OVERCOMING AUTOIMMUNITY

One Physician's Step by Step Journey to
Victory Over Her Chronic Illnesses

Karla Montague-Brown, M.D.

Cover design by: sam_designs1
Back cover author's photo by: Aaron Anderson

Printed in the United States of America

Dedication and Acknowledgements

There have been many individuals who have encouraged me on this journey.

I want to acknowledge and thank my family.

To my husband, Terrence Brown, thank you for honoring the vows we shared in 1986 to love in sickness and in health and for richer or poorer. We have experienced all of that and you have been there for me. I love you babe!

Thanks to Justin and Jordan Brown. I prayed to be a mother and God blessed me with you. You make me proud to be your mommy.

To my mother, Valeria Montague, I love you and thank you for your never-ending support. I'm blessed.

Thanks to my brothers, Glenn, Kevin, and Dewayne, for your love and encouragement through the years.

Lastly, I want to dedicate this book to the memory of my dad, Dr. Arnett Montague, who passed away in 2017. I'm grateful for his influence in my life.

CONTENTS

DISCLAIMER &
LEGAL NOTICE

AUTHOR'S NOTE

I am sharing my journey with autoimmune disorders in hopes that it will encourage and benefit others who may be struggling with similar issues.

We can take control of our health and make wise choices to help our bodies get well.

This book shares my personal testimony of overcoming auto-immunity. It is also my offering to encourage, empower, and equip others to take control of their health in order to live well.

It is my desire to help you achieve wellness from the CROWN of your head to the SOLE of your foot.

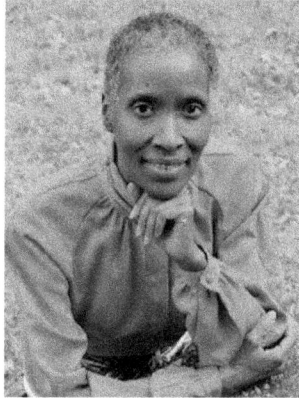

SECTION 1 - THE ILLNESSES

CHAPTER 1 – MY SYMPTOMS STARTING JANUARY 2019

It was the beginning of a new year—2019. I had been looking forward to 2019 and had shared with my business accountability partner, Shirah, some of my goals for the year, which included writing a book. My niece, Stacey, and her husband, Wayne, were coordinating an event for their work during the Dr. Martin Luther King, Jr. holiday weekend, and had asked me to come babysit their kids. I was happy to have the opportunity to bond with my great niece and nephews, and because Stacey and Wayne have three children (one of whom was a baby), I asked my son, Justin, to come with me to help keep them occupied. We had a great time with the kids from that Friday through Sunday. Yes, we were both tired from the activities of keeping up with three children ages one, four, and seven, but we enjoyed it.

A couple of days after we came back home, I woke up feeling achy with muscle soreness. It felt like I had been working out, but I really hadn't been doing any heavy exercise. I remember telling my husband, Terrence, "I don't know why my muscles are feeling sore, unless it's from picking up the baby this past weekend."

When we thought about it, we laughed, and he said, "Yeah, that's probably it."

I figured I would take some hot showers and I would be fine in a day or two. However, after a couple of days, it was not any better.

In fact, I'd started to feel worse. My muscles were sore all over, and I'd developed this overwhelming fatigue. I wasn't doing very much, but I was just so tired, stiff, and sore. *Do I have the flu?* I wondered. There were no cold symptoms, cough, or fever, but I couldn't figure out why I was so tired all the time. I was waking up tired. After taking my shower in the mornings, I would have to lie down and rest before getting dressed. Every joint and muscle from my neck down to my feet hurt. I was tired during the workday and tired when I got back home. My husband would have to help me get in and out of the car because I was so stiff and in so much pain. Normally, I take showers and my husband takes baths, but I found myself racing to get in the tub as soon as I got home from work so I could soak and turn on the water jets. The problem with this was that the heat would zap my energy, so even though the warm water felt good, I couldn't stay in long, because I always felt like I might pass out.

When I noticed that my joints and muscles felt swollen and tight and my skin was bruising for no reason, I knew it was time to go to the doctor to get checked out. Generally, I go to the doctor for my physicals, but unless I have a condition that appears to be lingering or worsening, I usually wait a while before making an appointment. These symptoms were all new to me, and because I am a physician, I knew something was wrong.

I work as a medical consultant with other physicians for the Social Security Disability department. My cubicle neighbor, Glenda, is an internal medicine physician, so I consulted her in what I call a "cubicle consult." We came up with a list of labs and studies for my primary care physician to investigate so we could figure out what was going on with me. Glenda, my primary care physician, and I had all been in medical school and residency together, and we are friends, so I knew my physician would not be offended if I came in with a list of what I thought should be done. She would just add to it or take away from it as she saw fit.

It was now time to call my doctor to make an appointment. Because we are close friends, I simply texted her cell phone. I still have the text in my phone, dated 2/4/19.

"Hey Carolyn, do you see walk-ins or work-ins? Or is it the nurse practitioner who does this? I've been hoping I would get better and not have to come back in so soon, but my body has been aching for the past two weeks and I don't know why. If I'm not better tomorrow I will probably call the office in the morning to see if I can get in. If I have to see the nurse practitioner that's fine as long as they consult with you at some point. You know how we are with our bodies. I'm starting to get scared because I'm not a sickly person, but I do realize I'm 57 now. You KNOW I've thought of the 'life-threatening possibilities' instead of the most likely scenarios. All the stuff I've tried to get better has not really worked except for temporarily. I feel like I've become 'OLD' in a matter of 2 weeks! This sucks!"

My sister doc came through for me and was able to see me two days later. She appreciated the list of lab tests I brought, and indeed, she added to it. I'm so thankful for her, and I praise God for any physician who listens, cares, and prays.

Because of my symptoms and swelling, I was offered the medication Prednisone, but I'm not one to take a lot of medication (I'll share more about why later). I declined to take it at that time and just really wanted to determine what the problem was so we could figure out how to best treat it. She understood my aversion to taking the medication, and we elected to wait until we got lab results back unless things got a lot worse in the intervening time.

Although I was in pain every day, swollen and stiff, I still had reason to have joy. Our family was in the process of buying a house. Even as I was questioning what was happening with my body and asking God to heal me, He was answering another prayer that my husband and I had been praying for a while as it related to purchasing a home. The day after my initial doctor's visit with my primary care physician, my husband and I were at the Title company signing papers for our new home. Yep, I was still sore and could barely move. I felt horrible physically and I just kept thinking, *Lord, we've prayed about this, and at this point I'm in so much pain I just have to trust you, because I'm just signing and wishing they would hurry up and be finished with all of these papers.* Finally, we signed the last document—thank you God!

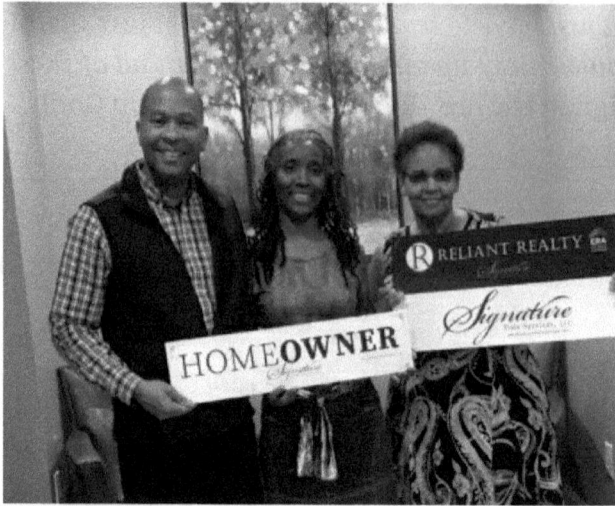

Terrence and I with our agent, Shalita. She helped
us realize an answer to prayer. I was achy, fatigued,
and stiff, but so very grateful!

CHAPTER 2 – THE SEARCH FOR A DIAGNOSIS AND DEALING WITH THE REALITY OF ILLNESS

A few days after visiting the doctor, I received a phone call from her. She informed me that they had received my lab results and then said, "We need to send you to a rheumatologist for further evaluation. It looks like you may have lupus or some other auto-immune disorder." My heart sank a little bit, because I knew that lupus could potentially cause a lot of different complications and affect different organs of the body. However, when I thought about my symptoms and saw my lab results, I was not surprised by what she told me.

I got in touch with the rheumatologist's office and was given an appointment for March 21, 2019—nearly six weeks away. I was thinking, *Well, I may be DEAD by then, but hopefully I'll be HEALED by that time and won't need to go at all.* Yes, I was praying regularly for God to heal me.

Remembering the story of the woman in the Bible who was healed when she touched the hem of Jesus's garment, I started telling God that I was touching the hem of His garment. I let him know that I had faith He could heal me right away. Although I wasn't really able to get on my knees to pray, I would lie flat on my back in the bed and move my hands around, trying to find the "hem of Jesus's garment." Each day, I would wake up still in pain, still swollen, stiff, and fatigued, and I finally figured out God had other plans for how He was going to heal me. It was like I could hear Him saying, "Baby girl, we ain't doing it like that this time . . . but I got you! Just trust Me."

My answer to Him would be, "Okay Lord, I will trust you. I just wanted you to know how I feel, and you said to ask You for what we need and want. I'm really not liking this being sick, but I'm trusting You to take care of me."

About a week or so after my initial office visit with my primary care doctor, I dragged myself to work. It was cold outside, and it took so much effort for me to just put one foot in front of the other. I wanted to stop and sit on a bench to rest, but I thought, *There's nobody out here to find me if something happens to me, so I'd better just get inside the building.* I finally got inside and to my cubicle and let Mary, the clerk in the cubicle beside mine, know that I was there but moving slowly. By the time I turned my computer on and sent my work schedule for the day to the printer, I realized I didn't have the strength or energy to even walk to the printer to retrieve my document.

My husband and I often text each other throughout the day, and he sent me a text shortly after I got to work to let me know he loved me. I texted him back, "I think I'm going home. I don't know if I'm just getting anxious or if something is wrong. I'm not in a whole lot of pain, but I'm just so tired. I'm not sure what to do. I'm scared."

We texted back and forth a little bit, and I asked him what he thought I should do. Finally, I said, "I think I may go to the hospital to make sure nothing is getting worse. I feel a little short of breath."

Well, my saying something about going to the hospital triggered him. He knew that was not my usual thing to do, so just the fact that I said that let him know it may be truly serious. He told me to go to the hospital and call my doctor when I got there. I was too afraid to drive, and the co-worker of whom we both thought to ask to take me hadn't arrived at work yet. I let Mary know what was going on, and because I felt like I couldn't get up to walk to anybody's car, I told her to call 911. To be clear, that is *so* not me. The last time (and only other time) I told someone to call 911 for me was many years ago after I had a bad reaction to some medication in the dentist's office and I thought I was about to die.

I didn't know what was happening with me this time, but I remember thinking, *I am NOT going to die up here in this cubicle at work.* I also remember wondering, *Is this how Daddy felt right before he died?* I ended up in the emergency room after being transported in an ambulance. My coworker, Becky, went to pick my husband up from work because I had the car at my job. They met me at the hospital. Fortunately, I did not have to be admitted, but they did do more testing to make sure my heart was okay and that I did not have any blood clots in my lungs. What a frightening and humbling experience!

During the six weeks while I was waiting to see the rheumatologist, I knew I had to do something to help myself in addition to praying, especially if I was trying to avoid medication. The changes in my body were so drastic I really couldn't avoid letting people around me know what was going on. Usually, I'm energetic, active, and involved in different activities. Yet in just a few weeks' time, I was moving slowly and not my usual self, continuing to rapidly lose weight, so I knew people could tell something was wrong. It was less stressful for me to just let people know that I was having some issues instead of letting them wonder or be hesitant to ask me if I was okay. I talked to my family, texted some of my friends, and shared with my church family, and because I have prayed for many people because of a Facebook post, I even shared it on Facebook.

There is a saying, "Much prayer, much power." I was soliciting much prayer on my behalf. I told some people, "Y'all say my *whole* name when you pray for me, so God will know which Karla you are talking about!" People added me to their prayer lists and prayer groups. Many people I didn't even know began praying for me.

In addition to praying, I started formulating a plan of attack. There is a scripture that says, "If my people, which are called by my name, shall humble themselves, and pray, and seek my face, and turn from their wicked ways; then will I hear from heaven, and will forgive their sin, and will heal their land." 2 Chronicles 7:14 (KJV). Now, I may not be using this scripture in the context of the chapter, but it became a go-to text for me concerning my illness. I am a Christian. I was surely being humbled. The prayer part was being covered. I was seeking the Lord's face [and the hem of His garment]. I needed to know from what "wicked ways" I had to turn.

As a health advocate and transformational speaker about wellness, I have tried to practice good health habits, but there is always room for improvement. Over the years, I have made changes to my diet. I try to rest appropriately, drink water, exercise, and think positively. It's not a perfect regimen, but I have been intentional about it. I came across this Facebook post from Jurne Azublah, a nutritionist, that stated, "You can't eat toxic foods and expect prayer to eliminate the toxins. You simply need to stop poisoning yourself."

My diet largely consisted of fruits, vegetables, beans, and nuts prior to my becoming ill, but because I don't like to cook, I felt like my "wicked ways" included commercially processed foods. Therefore, I made a conscious effort to eliminate—as much as possible—the commercially processed, "enriched" foods, and foods with preservatives and chemicals. Instead of canned, my beans and legumes now come dry from a bag. Most of my food comes from the produce section. My goal was to eliminate the foods that cause inflammation and increase the foods that combat inflammation.

In addition to the regular food I was eating, I started drinking what I call my "green drink." My oldest brother, Glenn, has a friend with experience with natural treatments, and that friend shared with me the ingredients for an anti-inflammatory drink. It consists of several different vegetables and spices to help with inflammation, so I was willing to try it. It does not taste great, but I drank it anyway. I didn't really know what I was doing when I made it initially, because I wasn't given specific instructions, just the ingredients to use. Over the months, I improved at making it. It still doesn't taste great, but I'm trying to live.

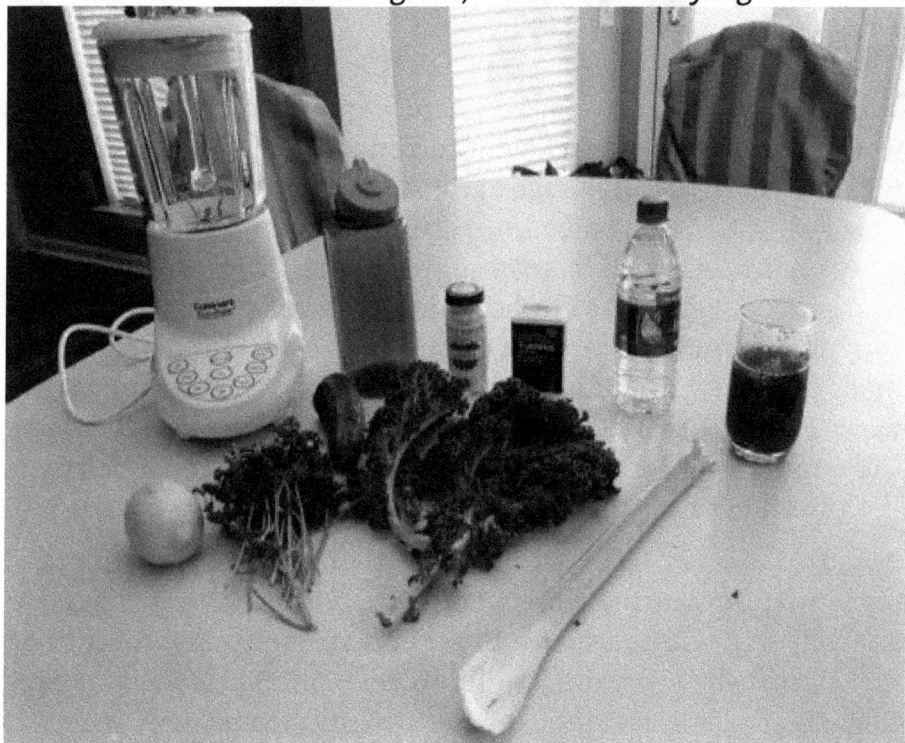

One day, my sons and I were in the kitchen and my older son, Justin, wondered what the green drink tasted like, so he decided to try it. After he poured out a little my younger son, Jordan, [who had NOT wanted to try it] chimed in, "It tastes like a lawnmower." I guess it was because it smelled like freshly cut grass.

We laughed, and Justin almost chickened out of trying it. I told him, "You ain't wasting my stuff I made. You better drink it and act like you like how lawnmower tastes!"

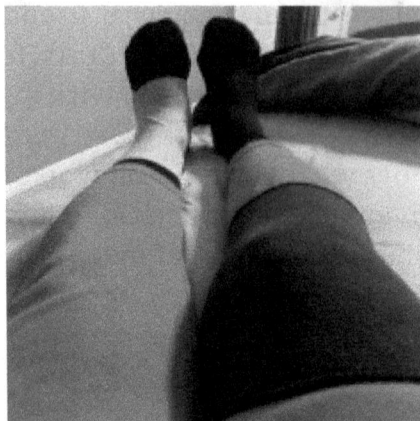

There were times in those first few weeks and months when I went to bed looking a "hot mess." One night, I had to literally laugh at myself, and even took a picture of how I went to bed. I had compression socks on both feet, an Ace wrap on my left ankle, a knee support on my right knee, and the heating pad right next to the bed.   If I'd had wrists and elbow supports, I would have worn them also. I even wondered if they made "all over the body" supports like the body suits snorkelers wear. My attire was not sexy at all, but it was all good. I was able to sleep and make it to work the next day without too much pain. I'm grateful to have a husband who loves me for me.

Because I was trying to get better without medication, I needed some help in figuring things out. I still didn't have a diagnosis and was still waiting to see the rheumatologist. My doctor had mentioned the possibility of lupus, so while I was not claiming that diagnosis, I decided to treat my symptoms as if that was what I had. I contacted several people I knew with lupus. I shared with them what was going on and asked for advice. One of those friends, Candice, is a young lady whom I met years ago when she was about seven years old. She is in her early thirties now and was diagnosed with Lupus when she was in her late teens or early twenties. She shared with me some of her journey and rec-ommended a book titled, *Goodbye Lupus – How a Medical Doctor*

Healed Herself Naturally with Supermarket Foods by Brooke Gold-ner, M.D. [1] I immediately purchased the book and began reading. It affirmed some of the things I was already doing, and I learned some other things I could do as well.

During the weeks when I was waiting to see the specialist, I was still in pain every day, and still tired. I was also dealing with the emotional ups and downs of not feeling well. I was continuing to lose weight, so my clothes were starting to not fit. My feet were still swollen, so I was wearing my rain boots every day (rain or sunshine). I remember posting on Facebook one day: *"I had already decided to wear my rain boots today even if the sun was shining because I'm scared my other shoes/boots won't fit or will aggravate my ankles. Anyway, I put my rain boots on (they were cute though) and*

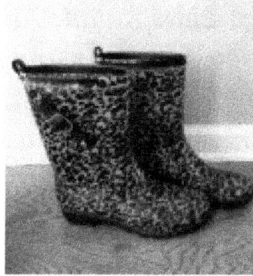

the sun was shining. *I didn't care what anyone thought either. But guess what! IT IS RAINING NOW!! LOL! So now I'm fashionable for the rain. I will bless the Lord at all times!"*

I had started writing a journal of my experiences and would share praise reports and progress updates on Facebook. This helped me emotionally, and I hope it was also an encouragement to others. One progress report that I shared which continues to touch me in a special way involved my anointing service. One Sabbath [Saturday] I approached one of the female elders at church and said, "Nat, if I had some oil, I would ask you to anoint me."

She immediately responded, "Karla, I was just thinking this week to offer you that service. When do you want to do it?"

My reply was, "Tomorrow!" We made an appointment for her to come to my house the very next day. I wrote the following Facebook post on February 24, 2019:

"I know many of you have been praying for me and I appreciate it sooooo much. I still don't have all the answers yet about what is causing my health challenges and everyday there seems to be something different to deal with but I remain encouraged. Sometimes I do get tearful and fearful but I try to intentionally not stay in that frame of mind because in the long run the fear robs me of my peace of mind. Adding to my frustration is that we are in the midst of a move and I just don't have the energy to help the "team" (my family) very much but it is getting done. I'm blessed to have a loving and supportive family. I'm also blessed with great friends, co-workers, and church family. Today I had a visit from my sister friend, Elder Natalie Adeleke, and she brought her anointing oils. Now, if you know her and me, y'all know we had "CHURCH" right up here in my house! Well, I wasn't quite dancing but if I could have y'all know I would have. Anyway, I just wanted to let you know that I am still praying for healing and still praising God for His blessings! I'm also lifting up others I know who are dealing with serious health challenges and bereavement. Please keep calling my name in prayer for my healing. I love you!" (Elder Natalie and I pictured together)

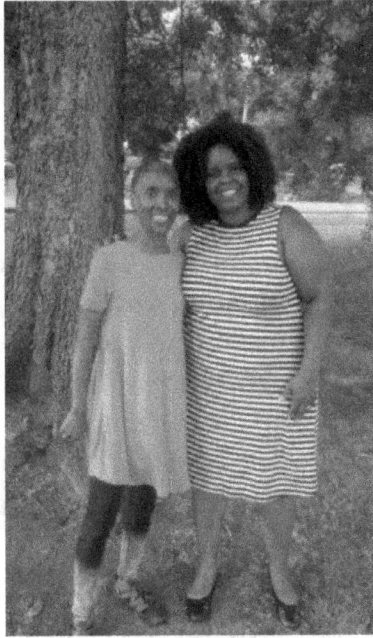

About a week later, I was finally able to wear some shoes other than my rain boots. I was able to graduate to tennis shoes. I needed the padding, because the soles of my feet hurt when I stood or walked. March 2, 2019, I was able to share another praise report on Facebook.

"Today is the first day since about January 20, 2019 that I have been largely pain free (at least for the past several hours). I went to bed last night with pain and stiffness all over my body after having had a good day. This morning I woke up with some pain, but I got ready for church. I was moving a little slowly and I wasn't ready when Terrence left so I rode with my sons. I thought I would wear my regular boots because the swelling in my foot seemed to have gone down...but I could only find one boot. (My family moved my stuff largely without my help because I wasn't able to help so I don't know where a lot of my stuff is). So, yeah...I wore the rain boots AGAIN. LOL! Anyway, I was able to sing with the choir, but I was afraid to move too much because I was scared that I would get short of breath or dizzy and I didn't want to pass out.

But it's kind of hard for me to be still when I sing, so I had to move a little bit. Y'all, let me tell you…it hit me… 'I'M NOT IN PAIN RIGHT NOW' and 'I'M ABLE TO WALK WITHOUT LIMPING!' Man, I just got so full. I've been praising God even through the pain, BUT when I realized I was pain free I was ready to dance for real. I probably did a little bit. I'm a crier too so y'all know I shed some tears and I don't have a problem shouting HALLELUJAH and PRAISE THE LORD either. I ain't even ashamed about letting y'all see me get a little emotional either. Anyway, I am just so excited that I'm walking sort of normally and without pain that I just had to let you know. I'm home now and still SHOUTING and CRYING (expressions of Joy and Gratefulness). Thanks for the prayers. Keep them going. One day I will tell more of the story. In the meantime, 'I will bless the Lord at all times. His praise shall continually be in my mouth.'"

Finally, March 21, 2019 rolled around—the day of my rheumatology appointment. My husband and I had been sharing a car and riding to work together, so we drove to his job first and then I proceeded to drive to the doctor's office from there. My appointment was for 9:20 a.m., but they wanted me to be there twenty minutes prior to get my paperwork processed. After I left Terrence's job, I calculated that I would get to the doctor's office about 8:50 a.m. —plenty of time to be on time.

When I was about two minutes away from the office, my car started losing power. I had no idea what was wrong with the car, but I knew it was getting ready to stop, and I was afraid that if I rolled into the intersection, I would not be able to make it completely through. I was thinking, *Really Satan, THIS is how you're going to do this?* Fortunately, I was at a stoplight and the signal turned red.

I quickly called my husband and told him what was going on. He told me to turn the car off and restart it. I turned the car off, but it would not restart. He said, "I will get an Uber ride and be right there." I tried not to panic, but I couldn't even remember where my hazard button was. I finally found it and turned the hazards on so the other drivers would know my car was having some issues.

I then called the doctor's office to let them know I was on their street, but my car had stopped. I told them I was just a couple of minutes away and that I would Uber there after my husband arrived to take care of our car. By the time my husband arrived, it was about 9:10 a.m. After I got in the Uber car and gave the driver the address, I was getting ready to call the doctor's office to let them know I was on my way.

They beat me to the call, ringing me at about 9:12 a.m. When I realized it was the doctor's office, I quickly let them know I was on my way and the GPS showed that I was two minutes away. However, the guy on the other end said, "I'm sorry, but you are going to be too late. You will need to reschedule. Do you want to reschedule now?" So much went through my mind in those few seconds before I told him, "No, I do NOT want to reschedule now." I was thinking, *I know it's not twenty minutes ahead of time, but I will still get there several minutes before my actual appointment time. Do you know how long I have waited for this appointment?* I didn't say all of that to him, but I did think, *If THIS is how you treat a new patient who just called you to let you know what's going on and you still tell me I'm too late when I would actually get there well before my appointment time, then maybe this is not the place I need to be.*

I knew I would not reschedule with them—I would just have to find another physician. I asked the Uber driver if he could take me home instead, which was about a twenty-five to thirty-minute drive away. He responded, "Ma'am, you've been through so much today, I will take you wherever you need to go." So, I went home! He felt that perhaps I should have gone to the doctor's office anyway and demanded to be seen, but I did not feel inspired to do that. I had been praying that God would lead me to the right physician. I told the Uber driver, "I'm thinking with my car stopping and with the way I was just treated that maybe that's not the place where God wanted me to be."

My mantra is, "I will bless the Lord at all times. His praise shall continually be in my mouth." So, while I was disappointed, I began praying and praising God for keeping me safe while I was in the middle of the street. I thanked Him for saving me from a potentially bad experience with a doctor who was not for me and let Him know I was trusting Him to lead me to the right place. I guess I needed a little more time to let my "natural remedies" work before having my lab studies repeated.

Throughout this experience, God showed me that He was still in charge. My car stopped at the stoplight and not in the middle of the intersection where cars were exiting the interstate. My husband was able to get to me within minutes. God even allowed me to have an "angel" experience. While I was sitting there in the street, there were no other people outside except for other drivers and a man to my right standing at the exit ramp of the interstate, panhandling. Suddenly, I heard a man to my left calling to the panhandler saying, "Hey man, I got five dollars for you if you come help me move this car." I have no idea where this man came from or how he ended up next to my car. I realized he was soliciting help to get me and my car out of the middle of the street. Even just reliving this experience, I start to cry.

They moved my car across the intersection to the parking lot of a business. This was just minutes before my husband arrived. Before I got in the Uber, I showed Terrence the man who was responsible for pushing the car out of the street and the panhandler. The man was standing at the corner. I told Terrence to make sure and thank him again. He said he would, but when I asked him about it later, he said, "Karla, I turned to put my stuff in the car, and when I turned back around the man was gone. He had just been standing at the corner, but then he just vanished. I looked across the street and down the street and couldn't find him. The pan-handler was back at his post, but I couldn't find the other man." So, it seems he disappeared just as mysteriously as how he appeared. I'm convinced he was an angel.

My new rheumatology appointment with my new doctor was scheduled for April 12, 2019. She reviewed my medical history and previous lab results and suspected there was some type of auto-immune disorder or disorders affecting me. She wanted to put me on a medication called Plaquenil, but after she told me all the potential side effects, I declined.

I explained to her my reluctance to take the medication for now, at least until we knew what was really going on. I'd had some bad reactions to medications in the past, to the point of ending up in the emergency room, so I tried to avoid new ones when I could. Because I let her know that my symptoms were improving some and the swelling was improving as well, she was willing to allow me to continue with what I was doing and just monitor me. She really wanted me to start the medication though.

My lab work was repeated, but they added more specialized tests that the primary care physician had not ordered. I'm happy to report that my results showed significant improvement. Some of the previously abnormal results were normal now, and the ones that weren't still showed significant improvement. For example, my initial ANA test, which was positive, showed a titer of 1:640. It had improved to a titer of 1:160 [low range would be 1:40–1:80]. The erythrocyte sedimentation rate went from 46 to 22 [normal range below 30]. I had some abnormalities on my x-rays, but not too severe. Thankfully, the results did not confirm lupus, but the abnormalities did indicate autoimmune disorders. I was given the diagnoses of Undifferentiated Connective Tissue Disorder (UCTD) and Inflammatory Arthritis. The physician stated that my condition could go into remission, it could stay the same, or it could progress to a specific disorder such as lupus. It was time for another update to my people. This is the text that I sent out:

"Finally getting some answers health wise. 2 main diagnoses: 1) Undifferentiated Connective Tissue Disorder; 2) Inflammatory Arthritis. NO lupus or Scleroderma or polymyositis at this point. #1 can progress to the other conditions or it can remain as is or reverse. So far, my labs were much better than the initial labs!!! YAAY! My Doc wanted to start me on some meds (which will take several months to kick in.) I wanted to wait on that since I am improving. I will expand on what I have been doing since it seems to be helping. She would prefer I start the meds

now but was willing to continue monitoring. I go back in 3 months. (So many potential side effects to the meds but I told her I would come back sooner or see my primary care if things worsened before 3 months) Keep praying!"

The July 2019 labs continued to show some improvement, but the November 2019 lab report really got me excited! Throughout the year, I'd continued to share some of my experience, my feelings, praise reports, and prayer requests. November called for a big praise report.

11/16/19: *"Thank you everyone for your continued prayers in my behalf. (Please continue the prayers). I could not wait to share this good news. Last week I told you I went back to the rheumatologist's office for follow up blood work. The nurse practitioner who examined me felt as though my joints were improving and she was very encouraging for me to keep doing what I had been doing. I have so far (for several reasons) elected to not start the medication the rheumatologist wanted me to start after my first visit in April. Because I told her that I was doing some things that I believed would help she agreed to monitor me without me taking the medication, but she preferred that I take the meds. In July my labs were improving or stable so she didn't push the meds as much but stated that she would repeat the BIG LABS at the November visit. At the November visit, the nurse practitioner advised me that if my ANA test (one of the lab markers) was still positive that they would really want me to start the medication. I didn't agree that I would, but I told her I understood. (Positive is generally not good in medical terms as it relates to test results). Anyway, I just saw an email regarding my lab results. MY ANA TEST RESULTS ARE…. (drum roll…) NEGATIVE!!! HALLELUJAH! PRAISE THE LORD! God is a HEALER! While I still have some concerns being investigated, I am praising God for what He has done and what He is doing and what He is going to do! So many of you have been praying for me and encouraging me I just had to let you know how I'm doing. I'm improving day by day. I give all the glory to GOD! I just had to stop and take a PRAISE BREAK! I love you all! #Iwillblessth-eLordatalltimes #Hispraiseshallcontinuallybeinmymouth*

CHAPTER 3 – DEALING WITH THE REALITY OF AUTOIMMUNE DISORDERS

Prior to being diagnosed with UCTD and Inflammatory Arthritis, I had been fairly healthy. Thirteen years prior, I was treated for a thyroid condition, which went into remission after about three months and no longer required medication after that point. I have continued to have my thyroid checked over the years and it has remained normal. The other conditions I've dealt with in the past were mainly cold or flu symptoms, sinus infections, or bladder infections. Those conditions generally only lasted a few days to a few weeks, and then I would be healthy again.

However, dealing with the diagnosis of chronic, auto-immune disorders has been a little scary. I was told and have read since: "There is no cure." The medications offered would not cure me, but hopefully they would modify my immune system or at least help with the pain and inflammation. The many potential side effects of the medications scared me. After speaking with co-workers, relatives, and friends who were dealing with similar conditions, it seemed that most of them had problems with the medications and had to be switched to others, with varying degrees of success. Some had to deal with adverse reactions to and side effects of the medications, and even though they were on the medications, they were continuing to have the symptoms of their illness on a regular basis.

Probably one of the most frightening things for me was that it seemed like every other day I was having different symptoms. Sometimes it would be overwhelming fatigue; other days my chest would hurt, causing me to lie down, or I would have abdominal pain. My eyes would do strange things as though something was happening with my eye muscles. I developed headaches. The pain would travel around. If I'd gone to the doctor every time I had a new or different symptom, I probably would have been at the doctor's office twice a week. I even developed a tremor in my hands. My family history includes multiple sclerosis, and I began to wonder if that was what I had. I did have a CT scan of my brain, which was normal at the time. In addition to the pain, fatigue, and other symptoms, I kept losing weight. I wondered, "Is this part of the UCTD, or is something else going on?" I began to wonder if I had cancer and it just hadn't been discovered. I lost about twenty-five pounds in a few months; however, I was not trying to lose weight.

The weight loss really concerned me. I've always been small, but I had finally as an adult made peace with my size, because I was healthy and muscular. However, I lost so much weight so quickly, including my muscle tone, that I felt like I looked sick. My clothes were too big, and I became very self-conscious about my appearance. I started to hate going places, because I didn't want people telling me I needed to gain weight or that I was losing weight [as if I didn't know that]. Thank God for a practical husband. When I commented about my clothes being too big, he said, "Well, let's just go buy you some clothes that fit." So, that's what we

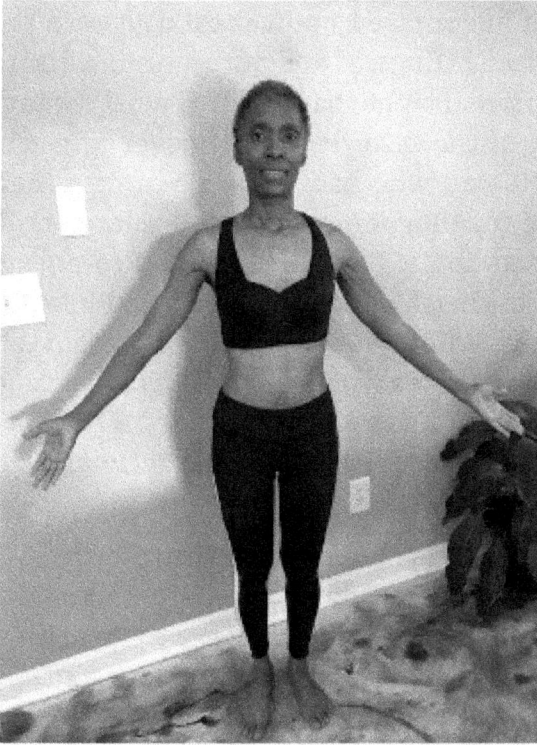

did. He also told me, "Just worry about gaining your health back. The weight will be what it will be."

One of the things that encouraged me was talking with people who were battling chronic illnesses and autoimmune disorders. That gave me a little more insight that much of what I was going through was just part of the disorder. I will never forget being approached by a gentleman who had read one of my Facebook posts. This was before my diagnoses, and I had related that my doctors were concerned about lupus. He wanted to encourage me and shared with me that his mother-in-law had been living with lupus for many years. He advised me to just pace myself. He said, "Karla, there will be times when you will feel pretty good, and then later you will just be tired, so just rest." That encounter meant so much to me, because that was exactly what I was experiencing.

My lab results have improved, and most are now normal—however, I have continued to not feel "normal." Some days, I wake up feeling great, but I'm learning I do indeed have to pace myself. I can do something as simple as fold clothes or cook a meal, and then I must lie down. And then at other times, I can walk around the block, go grocery shopping, do some cleaning and more, and be totally fine. It can be frustrating because my mind wants to do some things that my body is now not always able to do. During that first month or so, when I was really feeling bad, I was determined to attend a theatrical production for Black History Month, in which my sons were involved. They had worked so hard for months with the rehearsals, and I didn't want to miss their performances. My older son, Justin, was the music director and my younger son, Jordan, was one of the actors. It was held on a Saturday night, and I knew that I would have to take a nap during the day so that I would be able to make it. Fortunately, I was able to attend, and my pain was at a minimal level. I was one proud mama! However, several months later, I had to miss Justin's twenty-sixth birthday celebration because it was starting too late at night for me, and I knew it would end even later. I felt bad for missing it, but I had to honor my body. Thankfully, Justin understood.

It was wintertime when my symptoms began. The cold and rain really aggravated my condition, and it seemed as though I could never stay warm. My hands stayed icy, and I developed a condition called Raynaud's syndrome which causes pain in the fingers when they become cold. I began keeping gloves with me and would wear them even inside the house or other buildings. I felt like I looked stupid, but I began to not care what people thought [for the most part]. I even wore gloves in the summertime! When I knew fall weather and then winter were coming around again, I became a little concerned; however, I mentally prepared myself and knew to layer up when I had to deal with the elements.

When I think about how far I've come in the months since my initial symptoms and diagnoses, I realize I have much for which to be grateful . There was a time I could barely walk the few steps from the car to the house. Most of the time, I wouldn't even try to go upstairs in our house those first few months. Later, I was able to walk a few yards on my street at a slow pace, and then I progressed to being able to walk the neighborhood at a brisk pace. Hallelujah!

SECTION 2 - FEELINGS & MINDSET

CHAPTER 4 – "I WILL BLESS THE LORD AT ALL TIMES: HIS PRAISE SHALL CONTINUALLY BE IN MY MOUTH."

For several years now, I have adopted the mantra that is found in the Bible—Psalm 34:1, which says, "I will bless the Lord at all times: His praise shall continually be in my mouth." It's easy to praise God when things are going well, but when times get difficult, we sometimes get angry at God or question God. I am learning how to bless the Lord and praise Him, even when things get hard.

When several people close to me died, including my daddy, I had to learn to praise God for the lives they lived and how much their presence in my life was a blessing to me. I praised God that they were no longer suffering and that while they were living, they'd known that I loved them. This has helped me through the ongoing grieving process.

There have been many disappointments and frustrations on my journey, and times when I have been depressed, angry, fearful, and anxious, but giving God praise for who He is and remembering His blessings toward me helps to take the focus off of my problems and turn the focus on Him—the One who can solve my problems.

My perspective changes, and I am filled with an unexplainable peace. I realize it is the enemy of my soul, Satan, that seeks to cause destruction, while God allows the difficulties so I can learn to depend on Him. God comes through every time, even though I am often impatient and may want things done differently.

In early January of 2019, I chose a personal theme word for the year along with a song to help reinforce the theme. The word is "trust." I chose this before I became ill. After I became ill, I reflected on my theme and shared this post to my Facebook family on 2/11/19:

"At the beginning of the year I chose a personal theme word for the year and an inspirational song to encourage me with focusing on the chosen theme. My theme word is TRUST and the song I chose is "Trust in You" by Anthony Brown. Little did I know that just a few short weeks into January 2019 I would be faced with some major challenges that have caused me more and more to exercise my faith and trust in God. For the past several weeks my body's health has been under attack physically and often with the physical insults come anxiety and fear. Usually I'm on the other end of the health care dynamic and trying to assist someone else with their health needs. This time I'm the one in need of care. (Yes, doctors become ill also.) And yes, I have been to my doctor and testing is underway. Anyway, I have been praying daily for healing (even before we figure what's wrong with me.) I've been trying to "touch the hem of His garment and be made whole". I keep thinking, "Lord... what am I supposed to be learning during this time in my life's journey, and how do I bless someone else through this suffering?" Well, I don't have all of the answers but I'm reminded of a scripture that often comes to my mind in good and bad times: Psalm 34:1 'I will bless the Lord at all times: His praise shall continually be in my mouth'. So, I'm choosing to bless the Lord and praise Him. I'm choosing to walk in faith instead of fear. I'm choosing to allow God's grace to be sufficient for me this day! And I'm choosing to allow God's light to help me encourage and be a blessing to someone else by sharing this post. There have been soooo many times I have been encouraged by someone's Facebook post. I don't know who this post will bless but God knows who needs it right now."

I shared that post on a morning when I was struggling just to move, and during my personal devotional time, I read a passage from the book *Jesus Today* by Sarah Young,[2] which encouraged me and moved me to tears. I felt compelled to share encouragement with someone else who may be in pain [physically, emotionally, or spiritually]. Praising through the pain truly can help change a person's perspective, lessen the discomfort, and bring about healing.

About six weeks after sharing my personal theme and mantra with my Facebook family, I was able to share the following praise report on 3/30/19:

"#IwillblesstheLordatalltimes. I was able to make it to church again today and sing with the choir. I wasn't able to make it to choir rehearsal, but I was allowed to sing. I didn't stand every time the congregation stood because I was trying to make sure I could make it to the end of service without becoming overwhelmed with fatigue or shortness of breath. I'm grateful because not only did I make it through the service I was even able to speak during testimony time...I was able to stay for the fellowship meal. Last week when I went to church I had to pretty much go straight to the car when it was over. My stamina is improving. I debated with myself about posting this picture because I really don't like how I look these days but hey.... this is how I look these days. I asked my son to take my picture because when he saw me dressed for church the first thing he said was, "I like your shoes". I just looked at him and we started laughing and I had to give him a big hug. I nodded my head to him and said, 'YOU GET IT!' He said 'Yes.'"

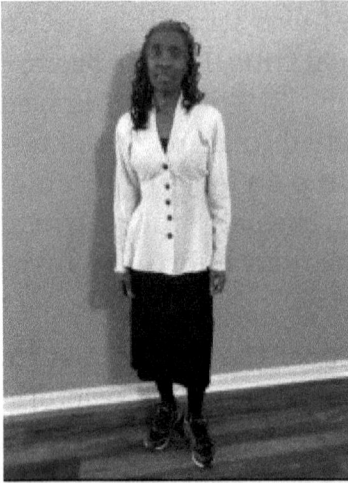

At that time, part of my pain included pain in the bottoms of my feet, which made it difficult for me to walk. So I had been wearing shoes that made it a bit easier. I had graduated from rain boots to tennis shoes. Normally, I would generally wear tennis shoes when I was taking a walk for exercise or for working out, but during this time I had started wearing them even when I went to work. Now, I'm no fashion queen, but I generally don't wear sneakers with my dress clothes. However, this week I had chosen to wear a dress skirt and blouse. I had my dark compression socks on, as well as some dark socks for more padding, along with a new pair of tennis shoes. I felt like I was trying my best but because of the weight loss, I felt like the outfit didn't fit quite right, and then on top of that the shoes... Anyway, Jordan's compliment warmed my heart, because he didn't say, "MOM, are you wearing THAT?" but instead just remarked that he liked my shoes. We had a big laugh.

My praise was: "1) I am here to even post a picture; 2) Jordan Brown helped me to laugh this morning; 3) I am in less pain today; 4) Even though I didn't think I was vain God is REALLY helping me to get over superficial vanity issues; 5) My family is so supportive; 6) Your prayers are working; 7) God is faithful; 8) Today has been a feel good day."

CHAPTER 5 – DEALING WITH THE FEAR OF DISABILITY AND DYING

After fifty-seven years of relatively good health, I found myself seriously ill. That realization was traumatic for me physically, emotionally, and spiritually. I was the physician whose job it was to help people get well. My passion has been sharing with others how to take control of their health and create lives of holistic wellness. I truly believe in—and for many years have been intentional about—trying to practice the principles that I teach others. While my efforts have not been perfect, I have tried to be consistent in implementation as I have continued to learn. *How did I get sick?* I wondered. *Now what do I do?* was my next thought. The big question though was, *Am I getting ready to die soon?*

There were times when I felt like I might die suddenly because I felt so bad. Other times, I felt like death would be a relief but, I did not want to die. I wanted to be well and be "myself" again. I was scared to die, because as messed up as things can be in this world, I had been enjoying life. No, my life has not been perfect, and I have problems just like everyone else, but at age fifty-seven, I was at a place where I had accomplished many of my goals and was for the most part past trying to prove myself to others. I had begun branching out in terms of pursuing my passion and what I felt God had been calling me to do at this time of my life and was excited about where God was leading me. After I got sick, I started feeling like I was really running out of time to do the things I had been wanting to do. "Lord, please give me more time," I pleaded with God. I thought about Hezekiah in the Bible, who asked God for more time and his life was extended for fifteen more years.[3] Of course, I didn't want to end up like Hezekiah and turn my back on God, so I let God know that too.

My other main concern in terms of why I was afraid to die was my family. When I got sick, my husband and I had been married for thirty-two years. I was thinking, *Man, we're in the zone now. We've been through ups and downs, had challenges and victories, and we are one. I'm not ready for him to be without me!* Full transparency, I also didn't like the thought of my husband potentially ending up with some crazy woman after my death. I also was concerned about my children. They are now young adults, but I feel like they still need me. What would they do if I died? I also wondered how my death would affect my mom and my siblings. Also, I didn't want to be forgotten.

One day, when I was stressing out and having a "meltdown," I remembered a prayer that I'd prayed when my sons were much younger. My husband and I were completing our wills and, we had to discuss who would care for our sons if we were to die while they were still minors. We agreed on a family member whom we asked to be responsible for them and who we felt would raise them similarly to how we were trying to raise them. However, every time I would think about someone else having to raise our boys, I would feel sad. I began to plead with God to keep us healthy and safe to raise our sons. I specifically remember asking God to at least let me live long enough to see my younger son graduate from high school and reach the age of eighteen. Jordan was probably about five or six years old at the time.

When I was having this "meltdown," I remembered that prayer. And then I thought, *Jordan graduated from high school in May of 2018. He turned eighteen in June of 2018, and I became ill in January of 2019.* "God, You KNOW I didn't mean it like that!" I prayed. I started renegotiating that long-ago prayer and said, "I didn't mean I wanted to die as soon as he turned eighteen. I think I said I wanted to live longer, but at least let me live to see them grown. Come on God, don't do this to me!" As I kept praying and calmed down, I also remembered my mantra, and I had to praise God that He had answered my prayer. My husband and I lived to see our sons become young adults. Thank you, God. I still have asked Him for more time, but I'm learning to leave the timing up to Him. I'm just trying to make sure I live in a way to maximize what God has given me and not sabotage myself or His efforts on my behalf.

Disability and/or the inability to make a living have also been big concerns. There have been some days I just couldn't do some of the things I wanted to do. *What if I have to quit working?* and *How will we have enough money?* were some of my questions.

I don't like being broke, and I became afraid of becoming disabled. I surely didn't want anyone to have to care for me, because I couldn't care for myself. Part of pacing myself meant scaling back my work hours. I had been working as a medical consultant for Social Security Disability and generally working four to five days a week.

In addition to that, I had launched my CROWN TO SOLE Wellness personal coaching and transformational speaking business about three years prior to my becoming ill. However, my energy levels became such that those hours and business activities became difficult for me to accomplish.

One day, I turned in my work schedule for the following month and had scheduled myself to work Monday through Friday each week. After I got home and thought about it, I realized I wouldn't be able to do that. The very next day, I told the clerk to tear up the schedule I had given her the previous day, because I had decided to start working three days a week to give myself time to rest and recuperate. I'm grateful I had the good sense to revamp my work schedule.

CHAPTER 6 – FIGHTING FOR HEALING AND GOOD QUALITY OF LIFE

Many days, I pray and ask God to help me feel normal. Sometimes I have felt like I would lose my mind because of the fear. Although my family knows that I'm not afraid to cry [especially tears of joy], I really don't like for them to see me feeling bad or fearful. I'm okay with letting my husband see it, but I feel bad when my sons see that I am feeling bad or afraid. There are times when it can't be helped, and I am not one to pretend.

One day, my older son Justin and I were in the kitchen. He asked me how I was feeling. Normally, I would have said, "I'm okay," but this time I really wasn't feeling okay. I was tired of feeling sick and tired of being scared. The tears started to flow, and I responded, "I'm just so tired of being sick—I want to be normal." He put his arms around me and held me, and then we were both crying. Sometimes you just need to let it out.

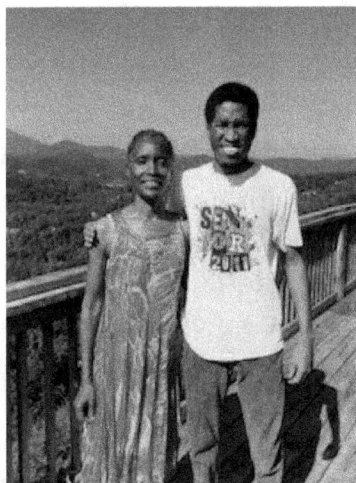

My older son, Justin and I

As my body and mind continued to be attacked, I strongly felt that my illness was not just an incidence of "Oh, this just happened." It was clear in my mind that the attacks on my health were due to spiritual warfare. Satan has been trying to end my life or silence my voice since I was an infant, as is evident to me by several situations I have encountered throughout the years. I believe that because I have intentionally decided to pursue the mission of sharing with others how to take control of their health in a way that honors God's temples [our bodies], Satan has become angry with me.

The thought occurred to me that God had allowed this illness so that I would learn to totally trust and depend on Him. However, I have also felt that this illness was not just for my benefit, but also for me to be even better equipped to help someone else. I began to pray, "Lord bless me and help me to be a blessing to someone else. Show me how to use my story and experience to help someone else and give You praise."

I really didn't know exactly the direction God was leading me, and I still had a lot of mindset issues that I needed to overcome. The mission of my CROWN TO SOLE Wellness business is to encourage, empower, and equip women to take control of their health and create lives of joy, abundance, and holistic wellness from the CROWN of the head to the SOLE of the foot. In other words, to create wellness of mind, body, and spirit.

Doubts began to creep in after I became ill, as I wondered, "Who will listen to me share about health and wellness principles if I'm sick?" My husband helped me to see my situation from a different perspective. He told me, "Karla, if you hadn't already been trying to practice those principles, you would probably be a lot worse off than you are. You could have become sick much sooner." He reminded me of how far I had come in just a few months, from barely being able to walk from the car to the house to being able to stroll around the neighborhood. He also reminded me that I had even started and was growing a garden. "You may be able to help people even more because of what you are dealing with." Then he said, "And you are still not on the medication!"

Terrence's words meant so much and helped me to regroup and recommit to the mission of fulfilling God's purpose for my life to assist others in practically achieving holistic wellness. My healing began with getting a handle on my mindset. This spiritual warfare needed to be dealt with spiritually before my emotional and physical healing could be accomplished.

At a recent family reunion in the summer of 2019, I spoke with a relative who had dealt with some major health challenges [cancer] who also believes in holistic/natural remedies and supernatural healing. We shared how our faith has been tested. During the conversation, she asked me, "Do you still believe what you have previously believed as it relates to healing principles?"

I answered, "I surely do!" The challenges, however, include learning what to do and then having the control and consistency to implement health principles that will build the body up instead of breaking it down.

CHAPTER 7 –
MY MINDSET
TRANSFORMATION

Many times, when someone has a chronic illness and is experiencing chronic pain and fatigue, they may develop depression or anxiety. There have been times I have dealt with both during this process [and even before my illness]. I hate being depressed. It's no fun waking up and dreading the day. I was raised in a Christian home, went to church regularly, and attended an elementary school sponsored by my church, so I had to memorize a lot of Biblical scripture.

As a child, I didn't realize how beneficial this would be for me later in life. Through the years, when I have become discouraged, sometimes I have awakened and just wanted to pull the covers over my head and not come out. However, it's hard for me to breathe like that, so I just come on out and deal with it. What makes it so bad though is I have a lot to be grateful for, so I wonder, "Why do I feel so bad?"

Some of those scriptures I learned many years ago as a child would pop into my mind when I needed them, even during those times when I was not regularly reading my Bible. When I became ill in late January and realized it was serious, I knew I needed a mindset transformation. I was scared, worried, depressed, confused, and maybe even angry at times, but that scripture kept coming back to me: "I will bless the Lord at all times: His praise shall continually be in my mouth." I would pray, "Lord you're gonna have to help me, because I'm really not feeling this right now."

I had read somewhere that negative emotions can negatively affect the immune system and contribute to illness, whereas positive emotions can help promote healing. Therefore, I needed to get my mind focused on positivity, even during the negative situations. Romans 12:2 (KJV) in the Bible tells us to "be ye transformed by the renewing of your mind." Another scripture that I have often shared with others is, "A merry heart doeth good like medicine: but a broken spirit drieth the bones." Proverbs 17:22 (KJV)

For me to start and sustain my healing process, I had to get my mind together. Because I believe my illness is part of the spiritual warfare, I decided to bombard and saturate my mind with scriptures to help renew my mind and jumpstart my healing transformation.

Many people focus on the negatives of our electronic devices and digital media [and they can indeed be used to cause harm], but I thank God for my gadgets even if I don't always know how to use them. For several months, I didn't always feel like reading, so sometimes I would just plug in my earbuds to my device and listen to the scriptures or the devotional. I searched for scriptures on trust, healing, anxiety, depression, and joy, and began to read and listen. I developed a list of scriptures to memorize and committed to learning a new scripture each week.

For my devotional readings, I downloaded the You Version Bible App and completed different plans that I felt would be helpful for me. The EGW Writings App is another free App that I use for scriptures, devotionals, and other inspirational readings.

YouTube has also been my friend. When I needed to listen to some inspirational music or meditations, that is where I turned. Gospel Artist, Yolanda Adams, has hit after hit, and so much of her music has ministered to me and helped to bring me up when I was down. There are many others, including Anthony Brown, Richard Smallwood, Tamela Mann, and DeWayne Woods, whose music has inspired me during my "stressing-out" moments.

Journaling has also been a source of therapy for renewing my mind. One of my mentors encourages her clients to journal positivity instead of just writing about complaints. So, while my journaling may contain some of my feelings, I've deliberately tried to turn them into prayers and talks with God.

I have learned that when the negative emotions pop up, if I dwell on them, they just snowball and I start to feel even worse. What I try to do instead is immediately start praying and recounting my blessings. The scripture Isaiah 26:3(KJV) states, "Thou wilt keep him in perfect peace, whose mind is stayed on thee: because he trusteth in thee." Refocusing my mind away from my fear and my problems and back on God's promises helps to bring me back to a peaceful state. Being able to share my feelings with health professionals who listen and share coping strategies has also been very valuable in dealing with the mental and emotional trauma associated with chronic illness.

CHAPTER 8 – ACCEPTING GOD'S WILL AND APPRECIATING LIFE MOMENT BY MOMENT.

One of the most difficult prayers I prayed was, "God, I accept Your Will for my life." That prayer did not come easy for me. That may sound strange coming from someone who is a Christian. I didn't realize how difficult it is to truly accept God's Will until I became ill and felt like I was dying. I did not want to die yet, but I also didn't know what God thought was best. If He thought it was "my time," I didn't want to pray "Your Will be done," because I felt like I would be giving God the impression that I was okay with dying, and I was not. I also felt like I would be giving up, yet I was fighting to get well. The fear and uncertainty would sometimes keep me awake. I was afraid to tell my husband how I was feeling, but I did, and he would encourage me to trust God. Sometimes he would just listen and hold me.

Finally, I had to "let go and let God have His way." While I still prayed for healing, I had to trust God to do it His way and in His time. It wasn't until I came to grips with surrendering my will that I started to have a sense of sustained peace. Yes, I still want to live and yes, sometimes the fear creeps in, but I keep giving it back to God for Him to handle.

Instead of waking up and dwelling on how much I dreaded to face the day, I started waking up and thanking God for letting me live to see another day. Gratitude became my focus as I realized that I had awakened and was still here. I now intentionally acknowledge being present and in the moment.

It has never been a problem for me to let my family know that I love them; however, it became even more important for me to share with my family and friends how much they mean to me and to regularly let them know I love them. We had two family reunions scheduled for July of 2019. My mother's family had planned a reunion and my husband's paternal family had planned a reunion. I wasn't sure I would be able to attend either. Because I wasn't sure how I would feel from day to day, I was somewhat reluctant to travel, especially without Terrence.

Fortunately, we only had to travel to my family reunion, as Terrence's family reunion was close to where we lived so we could stay at home. It was good to see everybody at both reunions, and my family was so supportive.

I had started feeling better, but I continued to feel somewhat fragile. I had to rest more than usual and be a spectator much of the time, but I was present! Many of my family members on both sides were aware of what I had been experiencing, and they had been praying for and encouraging me, so they were glad to see me. These reunions really emphasized for me how important it is to have a strong support system.

I remember being happy to see everyone, and I would greet each person with a big smile and hug. However, when I saw one of the cousins at my husband's family reunion, I immediately broke into tears.

We grew up in Memphis, Tennessee as childhood friends and became cousins when we married into the family. It's not that I wasn't happy to see Pam. Actually, I was overjoyed and overcome with emotion. Pam and her husband, Jonathan, had been dealing with some major health challenges in their family, which escalated shortly before I became ill.

However, Pam still found the time to reach beyond her own family's struggles and texted me almost every day for four months straight when she realized I was struggling. Her texts letting me know she was praying for me and inquiring about how I was feeling meant so much. I knew she was someone with whom I could be transparent. If I needed to cry or say I was scared, she would

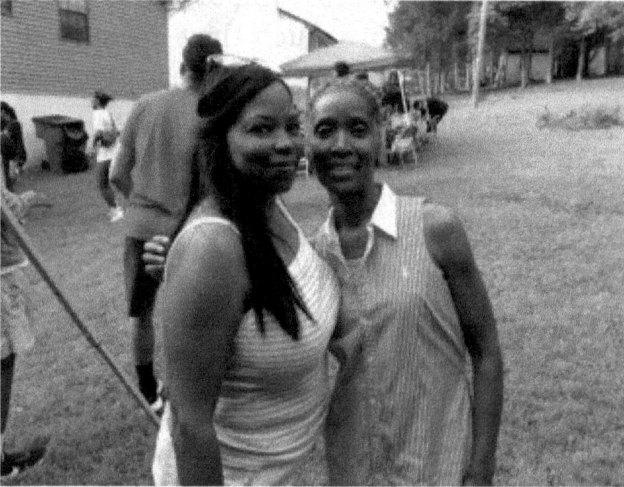

listen and not be judgmental. We had to take a moment and hug each other and let the tears flow.

(Pam and I at the Campbell Family Reunion)

Shortly after the family reunions, I experienced another boost to my healing. I was privileged to be one of the speakers at a "My Journey" event, where I shared with the audience some of my testimony and journey regarding chronic illness. This was the first time I had publicly spoken in a formal setting such as this about this phase of my journey.

What is so interesting about the invitation to speak is that it came at a time when I was still very ill. The coordinators of the event, Yvonne and Angela, knew I was ill and had a "bird's eye" view of what I was going through. They were witnesses to my decline, yet they asked me about a month or so after I became ill if I would be one of the speakers. I'm thinking, *the way I'm feeling, I don't even know if I will be here.* However, I answered, "Yes, if you guys have faith that I will be well enough by then, I guess I'd better get on board and have faith as well."

During the months leading up to the speaking engagement, I would start crying every time I thought about what I would share, because I kept thinking about how God was blessing me each day and helping me to improve. I started praying, "Lord, please don't let me start crying when I'm addressing the audience."

Now, I've already told you I'm a crier. So, I don't know what made me think I would get through that whole testimony without crying. Adding to the situation, my family [some of whom live out of town] showed up. My mother, Valeria, and all three of my brothers—Glenn, Kevin, and Dewayne—were present.

I knew my mother was coming but I didn't know that my brothers and sister-in-law, Fran, would be there. Other family members and friends showed up as well. Chile, I was crying before I even got up to speak, but God blessed, and I made it through.

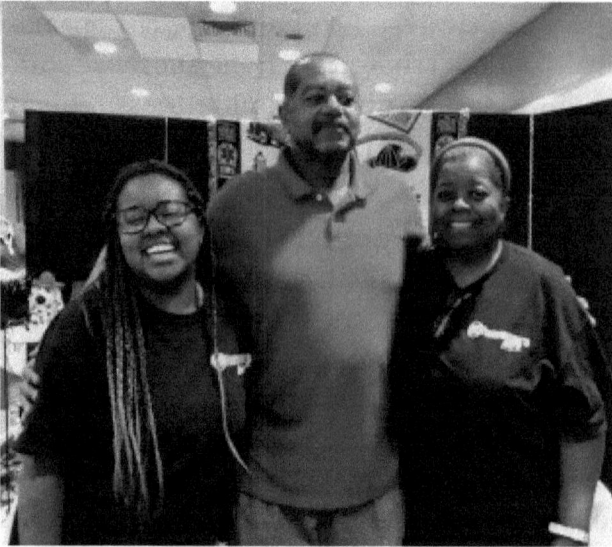

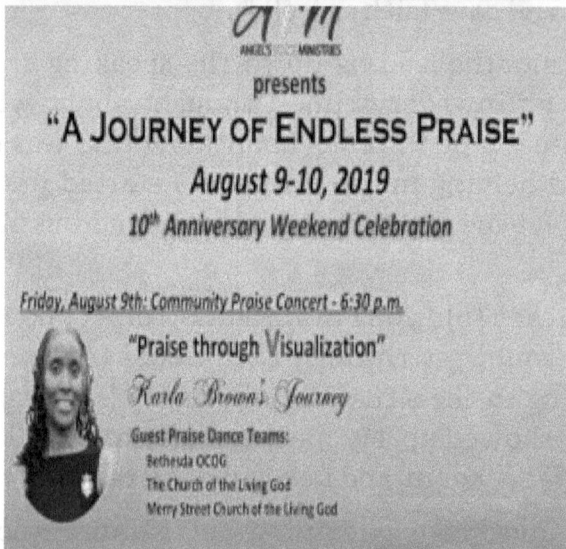

The Anderson family exercised faith by inviting me to
share "My Journey" long before I was better.

A couple of months after that, I had another speaking engagement
at a Women's event. I don't know if the event planner for this
event knew what I had been going through, but I was grateful for
the opportunity and praying that I would have the stamina to
endure, because it was an all-day event. About a week before the

event, I caught a cold and started losing my voice. I prayed that I would be well enough and that my voice would hold out. I remained well enough and my voice held out that day, even though it was gone the following day. I give God the glory.

I wanted to share about these two speaking engagements because the first one taught me more about faith, including the faith of others that I would get well. These engagements gave me something else positive to look forward to.

One of the things I worried about when I became ill was that my effectiveness as a transformational speaker would be diminished. However, God was showing me that instead of my voice being silenced, which is what I felt the enemy was trying to do, He was getting ready to use me in a more powerful way than He could have if I had not had afflictions of chronic illnesses.

If I am willing and trust God, then what the devil means for evil, God is able to use for my good and His Glory. I don't have all the answers as to where God is leading me or who I am supposed to bless, but I've given Him permission to use me how He wants to use me.

I choose to move forward in faith instead of fear. I'm thankful for each victory as they come and have chosen to use my personal and professional experiences to bless others to live a full and abundant life.

SECTION 3 – MY BACKGROUND: PERSONAL AND PROFESSIONAL

CHAPTER 9 – WHY I BECAME INTERESTED IN IMPROVING MY HEALTH

I was twenty-five years old and between my third and fourth years of medical school when Terrence and I got married. We knew we wanted children eventually, but not right away. Perhaps after two or three years of marriage, we would be ready. Well, after about three or four years, we felt ready, but it just didn't happen on our time schedule.

We were just at the point of thinking it was time to see a fertility specialist or consider adoption when I became pregnant. It wasn't until seven years after we had been married that we finally had our firstborn, a son we named Justin. I was thirty-two years old.

About four years later, we were excited to be expecting again; however, that pregnancy ended in a miscarriage. What a heartbreak that was! It wasn't until three years after the miscarriage that our second son, Jordan, was born. I was thirty-eight—he came a month before my thirty-ninth birthday. I had decided that if I hadn't had another baby by age forty, then Justin would probably be an only child.

Because I was an "older mom," I became more intentional about my health. Many of my friends and family members my age started having children about ten or more years before I did. I kept thinking, "Girl, you'd better take care of yourself so you can raise these boys." My family's medical history includes hypertension and diabetes, and I wanted to avoid these illnesses if I could. I didn't want my elementary-age boys to have to push me in a wheelchair because I had suffered a stroke or heart attack. So, I became more diligent about taking care of myself initially because of my children.

Later, as I more frequently started to see peers, friends, family members, and patients my age become ill, I became afraid of becoming ill myself. So, my "why" for my health transformation became more about fear of being sick.

As I began to mature spiritually, I reflected on the fact of my body being the temple of God, and how according to holy scriptures, I am of royalty as a daughter of the Most High. This paradigm shift in my thinking has been a major catalyst for my continued growth in taking care of mind, body, and spirit.

My "Why" progressed from living to make sure my boys had a healthy mommy, to focusing on fear of the pain and discomfort of illness, and finally to honoring God by taking care of this precious temple with which He has blessed me. I began to truly love me for who God made me to be, and to trust Him to help me live an abundant life.

It has made many of the challenges related to nutrition, exercise, and rest less of a struggle than they were previously. That's not to say that I don't still struggle, because I do. However, that mind shift has made a huge difference in why and how I do what I do or choose to not do.

CHAPTER 10 –
MY AVERSION TO
MEDICATION, AND
WHEN I LARGELY
STOPPED TAKING
MEDICATIONS

In 1998, I experienced one of the most frightening experiences in my life. The May 21, 2001 issue of the magazine *Medical Economics* published an article I wrote about the experience. It is titled "Visions of Death in the Dentist's Chair." The article recounts my office visit for a routine dental appointment to have some teeth fillings. When I was a child, my mom would take us to the dentist for regular check-ups, and as a young adult, I had my wisdom teeth pulled, so I was familiar with the routine.

My appointment was scheduled for after work, and the dentist's office was in the same complex as the medical practice where I worked. I was only a little worried about the pain from the needle stick to inject the local anesthetic and then I would be fine I thought. I expected the familiar numb-lip feeling after the injection; however, things quickly escalated to something more. My face felt flushed and warm, and I became somewhat uncomfortable. The assistant in the room with me must have sensed my discomfort and asked me if I was okay. "I'm feeling kind of warm," I replied.

Shortly thereafter, I began to get drowsy and the left side of my body began to tingle. That was strange to me, and I became a little more concerned. I asked the assistant if the medication was supposed to make me sleepy. When the dentist came back into the room and saw my expression, he asked whether I was okay. "I'm not sure," I told him. I tried to explain what I was feeling. Then my head started to hurt, feeling like it would explode. I felt off balance and in a state of mental fog. It took extra effort for me to breathe, and I had to think, *inhale, exhale.* "Help me!" I cried out. I was terrified. I was generally the cool, calm, collected and don't let them see you sweat type, but now my composure was gone.

I got up to walk around to see if that would relax me, but I started to feel like I was going to pass out. When I passed a mirror, I found it odd to see my reflection. I didn't know if I was losing my mind, but I felt like if I passed out, I was not going to wake up. *I'm going to die*, I thought. Full-blown panic struck!

"Call 911," I instructed the dental staff as if it were my medical practice. I wanted the paramedics there and ready to intubate and resuscitate me if I stopped breathing, because it was taking so much effort to breathe. I was transported to the ER, and it was determined that the local anesthetic, Carbocaine, had likely entered by bloodstream and caused the reactions I'd experienced. Whatever the problem was, the experience helped me to have a greater respect for the medications I had been prescribing for my patients. Although I would still take medication if needed, I became a bit more hesitant to take something I had not previously taken.

Several years after this experience, I started noticing side effects or adverse reactions to medications I had taken previously without problems. This made me even more leery of taking prescribed medications or even over-the-counter ones. I used to keep medications like ibuprofen, acetaminophen, and cold medications in the house for fevers, aches, pains, and cold symptoms, but I started noticing some issues even with these.

Another concern for me as a medical professional was the issue of "poly pharmacy," which refers to the use of multiple medications to treat one or more medical conditions in a single patient. I had quite a few patients on multiple medications for different ailments, and I would always become concerned if I had to prescribe another medication, even if I felt it may be needed. The list of side effects for one medication is often long, and then to add other drugs makes it difficult sometimes to tell if the ailments experienced are due to the side effects or interactions of the medications.

Please, don't misunderstand me. I am NOT saying that people should never take medications. I'm not even saying that I never have or never will take medications. They are often helpful, especially if one is not aware of other things that can be done to help combat or reverse illness. However, I do believe that we can have better control of our health and avoid so many medications and the associated bad side effects if we can learn and adopt certain health principles and other methods to prevent and treat illness.

When I first began my medical practice, I read a book called *Ministry of Healing* written by Ellen White.[4] It is not a traditional medicine book, but it contains valuable principles to help individuals prevent or control many lifestyle-related medical conditions and illnesses.

Over the years, I have read other publications and attended workshops and seminars designed to promote lifestyle principles for optimal health. As I began to incorporate these principles as part of my lifestyle, I would try to share with my patients in order to maximize the effects of the traditional medical treatments offered.

Often, there was not much interest in making drastic lifestyle changes, because it can be hard to do and maintain. I have had patients tell me, "Doc, can you just give me another pill or increase my dose?" when I would counsel them about their nutrition as it related to treating their diabetes or other conditions. However, there were patients who were interested in what they could do in addition to or instead of medication to manage their disease.

As my interest in natural remedies for healing grew, I continued to seek out opportunities to learn and expand my knowledge base. My home library contains many books dealing with natural remedies for healing.

In 2011, I enrolled in a course for natural healing, which assisted me in making the decision to avoid medications as much as possible. It's kind of difficult to make that decision when you don't know what else to do to treat illness.

As I began to make more changes in my lifestyle, especially as it related to the foods I chose to eat, I noticed that I generally didn't need the medications that I used to need. My sinus problems weren't as severe as previously, I wasn't developing bladder infections as often, and I was able to treat pain without resorting to ibuprofen or acetaminophen.

CHAPTER 11 – MY JOURNEY TO A WHOLE FOOD, PLANT-BASED DIET

My lifestyle journey has been one of continual progression, and I realize that it will continue to be a work in progress. For example, I grew up not eating pork and certain types of seafood; however, I did eat other meats like chicken, turkey, beef, and some fish. I also ate eggs and sometimes drank cow's milk which I did not like. Hamburgers and cheeseburgers were my favorite meat dishes. My mom's meatloaf was also a dish I enjoyed. I loved glazed donuts, brownies, Snickers bars, and lemon cake. Because I don't like to cook, I have also had my share of fast-food and restaurant meals.

When I initially decided to stop eating meat for preventive health reasons, I discontinued the beef first. I felt like chicken and fish were fine and healthy for me. However, I got tired of hearing about the salmonella outbreaks due to chicken [yes, I know that vegetables and fruit can have issues, but I was hearing more horror stories about the chicken]. So, I made the decision to stop eating it. One of my friends has a daughter who was about nine or ten years old when she decided she wanted to be a vegetarian. Nobody else in the household was a vegetarian, but I watched this girl for a whole year as she avoided eating meat. I was so impressed and decided if this ten-year-old girl could make that decision and stick with it, surely, I could give up chicken and poultry. That was in the mid-1990s.

It wasn't until 2011 that I finally decided to adopt a plant-based diet and stopped eating fish and dairy products. I'm sure there were probably times when there may have been dairy in something I ate if I didn't cook it myself. It has been a challenge, but with the progression of my mindset and my "why," it is probably not as difficult as it could be. As I mentioned previously, I was always healthy up until January of 2019. The attacks on my body seemed to come from nowhere. As a matter of fact, a few days before I became ill, I wrote an entry in my gratitude journal that I was grateful for good health. I was feeling good, and then all of a sudden, I was feeling horrible on a regular basis. When my symptoms and lab results pointed to an auto-immune disorder as the likely culprit, I was thrown for a loop. Here I was trying to avoid hypertension, diabetes, and high cholesterol, but then I was knocked on my back by my body attacking itself!

I still believed in the healthy lifestyle principles that I had adopted and been promoting, but I needed to know how to maximize these strategies. Inflammation was a major factor in my conditions, so I needed to figure out what else I could do to combat the inflammation. I had been dragging my feet with moving forward to the next step of my nutrition journey goals. One of my goals prior to my becoming ill was to eliminate as much as possible the heavily processed foods from my diet as well as fast-food meals. Although I wasn't eating a lot from fast-food restaurants, I was still eating processed foods, because it's so convenient, and as I mentioned before, I HATE to cook.

Well, now it was time for me to go ahead and eliminate the processed foods as much as possible. If the ingredients listed something other than the food I was purchasing, such as additives, chemicals, several oils, etc., I would avoid it.

Most of my time in the grocery store began to be spent in the produce section and the area for the spices and herbs. I still don't like to cook, but I like to live, so I do what I have to do. I have adopted what I consider to be an anti-inflammatory diet. While I still have some health challenges, I have come a long way. It's not always easy, but I don't want to go back to how I felt during the first half of 2019.

CHAPTER 12 – MY HEALTH CAREER AS A PHYSICIAN

"What do you want to be when you grow up?" is a question that children are often asked. My answer from the time I was about ten or eleven years old was usually, "A doctor." I didn't really know any medical doctors personally at that time, and my first role model for the type of physician I wanted to be wasn't even a real doctor. He played one on television. Yep, I LOVED Marcus Welby, MD!

Marcus Welby, M.D. was a television series broadcast from 1969 to 1976. Dr. Welby looked nothing like me, nor did he physically look like most of the men I knew personally. I grew up in a largely African American environment. During my early upbringing, most of my world in "real life" was surrounded by black people. I would see Caucasians and people of other races on television or when we would go places, and my parents interacted with a few, usually for business purposes, but the people I knew up close and personally mostly looked like me. However, on television, I saw very few African Americans when I was a child. So, we watched what was on, and somehow, I got hooked on Dr. Marcus Welby. He was so kind, smart, and patient, and it seemed that in thirty minutes each week he would "heal the world." I wanted to be like that.

Later, in the early- to mid-seventies, I found another role model in the person of a college student named Donna Willis. She was one of the daughters of my childhood pastor and was attending college as a pre-med student. When she learned that I wanted to be a doctor, she took me under her wing [even though she wasn't a doctor yet]. Whenever she would come home on break, she would ask me, "Are you still planning to be a doctor? How are you doing in school?" She would encourage me to "hang in there." She eventually went to medical school and earned her medical degree as a physician. Her encouragement was so motivational for me, especially when I finally went away to college [where most of the people did NOT look like me] and my college advisor [who looked somewhat like Marcus Welby] tried to convince me to change my major. I got the impression he felt like I "didn't belong" at this elite institution and that I wasn't "good enough." I felt so humiliated sitting there in his office and wanted to cry, but I was determined that he was NOT going to see me cry. I just thanked him for his time and left his office. No, I don't think I ever went back to see him, not even years later when I eventually earned my medical degree.

After a couple of years in college, I transferred schools from a fairly large university to a small college in Huntsville, Alabama: Oakwood College [now Oakwood University]. While I enjoyed much of my experience at the larger university, I sometimes felt invisible and unwanted by the masses. My sense of rejection led to a period of discouragement.

When I transferred schools, the difference in the atmosphere was immediately noticeable. Oakwood is a historically black institution of higher learning. There were many people who looked like me, and I was immediately embraced and included. I transferred in the middle of the school year and I thought everybody would already have their friends and maybe I would be left out. I was wrong. I found study partners and mentors and was included in study groups. The professors seemed to really care and got to know the students. Instead of the "every man for himself" mentality, the thinking was, "We're going to do this!" The pre-med students referred to each other as "Doctor." When I received my acceptance to medical school, my roommate and fellow students seemed to be just as excited as I was.

I learned from my earlier experiences how important it is to have role models and mentors and how valuable it is to be affirmed. I also realize that I must pay it forward and be a role model and mentor for someone else. There is a teenager in my church, Atheia, whom I discovered a few years ago wants to be a physician. When she told me this, it immediately took me back to what Donna Willis had done for me many years

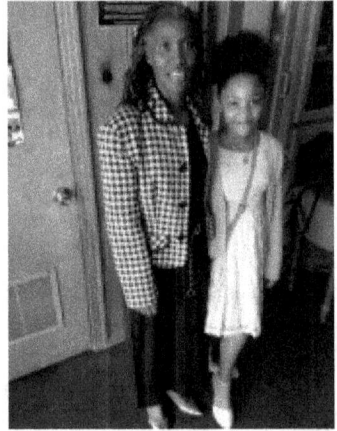

ago, when I was about the same age.

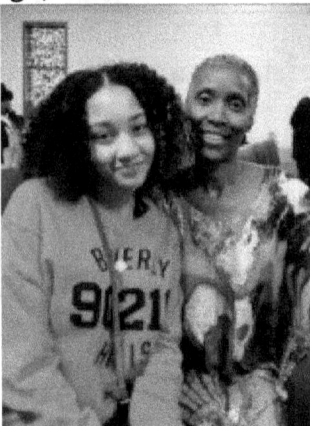

I took her under my wing, and for the past several years I have intentionally tried to encourage her on her journey.

Upon graduating from undergraduate school with a degree in

Biology, I entered Meharry Medical College in Nashville, Tennessee the following semester. Medical school was NOT easy, and I had my share of challenges along the way. However, it was also during this time that I met Terrence, the love of my life. We got married between my junior and senior years of medical school. We picked our wedding date based on when I would have a break in school. I wanted to make sure we had a honeymoon! In May of 1987, my dream of becoming a physician became a reality as I received the degree of Doctor of Medicine. My residency in Family Medicine was completed three years later. For almost twenty years after I completed my residency, I took care of a variety of patients of all ages as a Board-Certified Family Physician. In 2009, I transitioned from the primary care setting and became a State Agency Medical Consultant for the State of Tennessee Disability Determination Services.

In addition to seeing patients, I have had many opportunities for speaking engagements, especially regarding health and wellness. The first time I was asked to speak for a health seminar, I was a new, young physician. A member of my church, Gwen Brown, asked me to speak to the women's group about women's health concerns. I was afraid to accept the invitation and told her to let me think about it. Who *is going to listen to me?* I wondered. My fears had me asking myself, *What will I say and what if they are bored? What if they ask questions I can't answer?* At that time, I was somewhat quiet and unsure if this was something I could do. I shared with one of my medical colleagues, Larry, that I had been asked to speak and wasn't sure if I could do it. He said, "Karla, you have to do it."

My attitude started rising, and I asked him, "What do you mean I have to do it?"

Larry simply smiled at me and quietly said, "There will be people who will listen to you because of your position. You have to give back." That stopped me in my tracks. I hadn't thought of it like that. I was convinced and told Mrs. Brown that I would speak for the women's group. What a wonderful experience I had speaking to the ladies. I didn't know that I would enjoy it as much as I did. After that experience I decided that if someone needed me to speak and I was able to do it, then I would do so as much as possible.

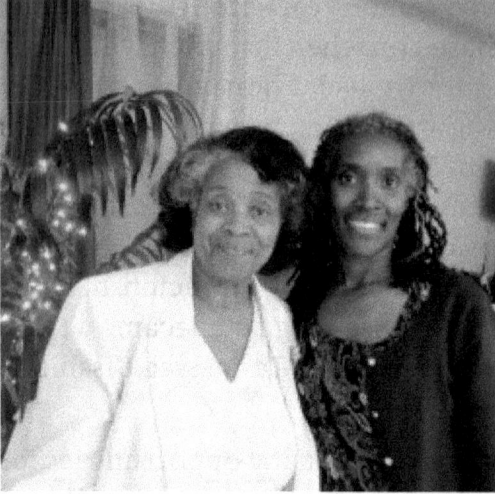

I owe a debt of gratitude to Mrs. Gwen Brown. Almost thirty years ago she extended to me my first invitation to speak/conduct a workshop as a health care professional. I have accepted many speaking engagements since that time.

SECTION 4 – SHARING TO HELP OTHERS

CHAPTER 13 – MY JOURNEY TO TRANSFORMATIONAL SPEAKING AND WELLNESS COACHING

Early on in my medical practice as a new physician, I would counsel my patients about lifestyle behaviors for wellness, but it later it hit me that just telling people to "eat a well-balanced, healthful diet" or "drink more water" was not really giving them much to go on. As I learned more for myself about creating my own lifestyle for health and wellness, I realized I was not giving my patients the tools regarding how to make changes and what to do. It's not always easy to make changes and stick with the plan. I learned this from my own personal journey.

The more I cared for patients in the primary care setting and prescribed more medications, the greater my desire became to motivate, encourage, and teach others how to live in a way designed to help them heal or prevent illness. Although I realized the need to treat patients for where they were as it related to their illnesses and lifestyles, I became dissatisfied with prescribing more and more medications without being able to fully educate and help my patients take control of their choices for health. Each medication, even though it may be designed to treat a certain condition, has its own potential side effects. Then, as I've described, you must worry about the interactions between them if a person is on more than one medication. Don't get me wrong, sometimes it is necessary to treat with medications, but too often we end up treating a lot of symptoms and then causing other symptoms or conditions that need to be treated.

Also, there are many who don't want to make changes or who struggle with making changes, but you still must do the best you can to help the patient live. I'm reminded of one of my patients who was a very heavy cigarette smoker. He was a kind gentleman whose appointments were at the end of the day after he left work. I was treating him for hypertension, high cholesterol, and severely elevated triglycerides. Before he would come to the back to the treatment rooms, I would know when he arrived in the office because of the smell of cigarette smoke. At each visit every few months I would encourage him to quit smoking because it would help control his blood pressure, cholesterol, and triglycerides. I also warned him about the potential danger of lung cancer. After a few years, he finally told me in a respectful, quiet voice, "Doc, I don't want to stop smoking."

I just had to laugh inwardly at myself, as I smiled at him and said, "Oh, okay ... but if you ever change your mind and need help, just let me know." I had been trying to do my job and "save" him, and he was quite comfortable with the way things were. Of course, I made a record of that conversation in the chart and continued to see him every three to four months to renew his prescriptions. I left him alone about smoking cessation, and we got along just fine!

However, there are many who would like to make lifestyle changes, but don't know exactly what to do. My dad and I had a conversation about a year or two before he died. He was being treated for several conditions and was being prescribed more and more medications.

My brothers, my mom, and I were concerned about the number of medications. Many of the symptoms he was being treated for also seemed to be side effects of some of what he was taking. He finally said to me, "I know I'm on too much medication, but I don't know what else to do." That was what I had been waiting for—for him to realize the need to make some changes and seek help. As a family, we worked together to help him make some lifestyle behavioral changes, and I believe it helped him to have a better quality of life his last couple of years than he'd had in the few years prior to these changes.

My medical consultant services with the State of Tennessee Disability Determination Services has given me an even greater view of the consequences of lifestyle choices. Every day when I go to work, I review the medical records of individuals applying for disability benefits. While there are many conditions that may be congenital or have an undetermined cause, there are also many conditions that have affected the applicants and caused their disability due to unhealthful lifestyle choices.

Over the years, I have been approached by individuals wondering what they could do to lose weight, or control their blood pressure, diabetes, or some other chronic condition. I always want to help and give sound advice that will be of benefit and do no harm. Working as a medical consultant for the State of Tennessee has given me more flexibility to accept more speaking engagements to facilitate workshops, seminars, and deliver keynote addresses. Several years ago, I started developing a plan to help individuals, especially women, take control of their lives and adopt healthful lifestyle behaviors to achieve optimal wellness.

In 2015, I took a huge leap of faith and launched my business, CROWN TO SOLE Wellness. Through transformational speaking and wellness coaching, I encourage individuals to take control of their health and well-being by providing trustworthy, practical lifestyle strategies to achieve lives of joy, fulfillment, and holistic wellness. My goal is to use my professional and personal experiences to encourage, empower and equip individuals to make practical, doable lifestyle changes so that trying to be healthy is not seen as a drudgery or form of punishment.

I've reached a point in my life where happiness and success go beyond just financial or career achievements. We get to a point where we want to be fulfilled and enjoy life, but we've been busy raising kids, working on a job, involved in church or civic activities, and developing relationships. These are all good, but one day we realize that we have been so busy taking care of everybody else that we have neglected ourselves. Our health and happiness suffer.

Perhaps you can relate to the lady who approached me for help after I had given a health talk at a women's conference. She had been struggling with obesity all her life and had developed high blood pressure, diabetes, and arthritis. Her son was now a young adult, and she was at the point of being able to retire in a few years. She was discouraged, felt like giving up, and worried that she would not be able to enjoy her retirement because of poor health. Her medications were not making her better, and she didn't know how to help herself.

Maybe you can resonate with the story of the young single mom with several school-aged children who sat next to me and asked for help losing weight. She was struggling with issues of low self-esteem and couldn't figure out how she could lose weight.

You possibly can relate to how I have felt at times, tired of waking up, and instead of being excited about the day, you want to pull the covers up over your head and not come out to face it. I started learning and incorporating certain lifestyle principles initially to avoid hypertension, diabetes, obesity, arthritis, and other chronic illness. However, I have discovered that these same principles have helped me deal with depression and anxiety. Now that I have developed auto-immune disorders and my body has started attacking itself, I have used these same principles to help me cope with these health challenges and to help reverse some of the effects.

When I first became ill in early 2019, I was convinced it was part of a spiritual attack to discourage me and to keep me from helping others. My experience has drawn me closer to the Creator of the Universe, and I understand that my experience is not just for me, but rather that my purpose is to continue to use my gifts to be a blessing to someone else as it relates to holistic wellness. I have developed a greater capacity for compassion for others, and I understand firsthand chronic pain, overwhelming fatigue, and fear of the unknown.

I don't know how long my journey will be on this earth, but I'm determined to make the best of it and to help others create a lifestyle plan to move from simply surviving to thriving. Each day, I commit to taking control of my life to pursue wellness from the CROWN of my head TO the SOLE of my foot. In other words, I'm striving for wellness of mind, body, and spirit. You can do the same.

CHAPTER 14 – CROWN TO SOLE WELLNESS

One of my frustrations when I was seeing patients as a family physician was my concern of wanting to do more to educate patients as it relates to holistic wellness. My journey is a process of continuing education and efforts to implement what I learn.

When I truly embraced the ideas that my body is the "Temple of God" and that I am a daughter of the Most High I realized that I am of Royalty. My desire is to care for God's Temple and live like the Royalty I was created to be. My mission is to help others do the same.

People don't always realize that they can have some control over their health and well-being. We may not be able to control everything, but we don't have to just roll over and take whatever comes our way. I want to share with you some guiding principles that I have adopted for myself and that I teach to others based on my years of professional and personal research and learning.

These principles are what I call: Eleven Steps to CROWN TO SOLE Wellness. CROWN TO SOLE is also an acronym to help you remember the principles as you transform to create your lifestyle of wellness.

"C" represents CONTROL. Exercise Self-Control. We have control over the choices we make; however, it often requires discipline to make wise choices. It helps to remember your "why" when it comes to making difficult lifestyle choices. The consequences are heavily dependent on the choices we make.

My husband and I have two sons who are now young adults. When they were very young, my husband began regularly advising them: "Learn to discipline yourself now, so that someone else won't have to do it for you later." That's good advice for all of us. When our younger son, Jordan, was in kindergarten, his teacher's classroom theme was "Candyland." On Fridays, there would be a special treat for those whose behavior had shown wise choices in following the classroom rules from Monday through Thursday of that week. The treat might be to watch a movie or eat popcorn or something else not usually done every day. Friday was called "Sweet Friday." Jordan was disappointed week after week, because he couldn't quite make all the right choices from Monday through Thursday, so he couldn't participate in Sweet Friday. Week after week, his teacher, Mrs. Edmond, and I would encourage him.

One day I asked him, "Jordan, did you make it to Sweet Friday this week?" With sadness in his voice, he replied, "No. Mommy, I try to make good choices, but sometimes I mess up."

I couldn't even be mad at him. I told him, "Baby, I understand. Sometimes I mess up too. We will just have to try harder tomorrow, Okay?" One day I was at work and received a phone call from Jordan, who was on his way home from school with his dad. He was so excited. "Mommy guess what?" he hollered into the phone. "I made Sweet Friday today!" He was happy and so was I. I was so proud of him.

Jordan's experience shows us that even though we mess up sometimes, we shouldn't give up on trying to reach for the prize. We are bound to hit the target eventually. Now, I can't say that he made Sweet Friday every week after, but we did celebrate the "wins." I encourage you to stick with the process and celebrate your victories.

"R" reminds us to REST. Our bodies need regular rest periods for maximum health benefits. Sleep deprivation is detrimental to physical and mental well-being. Proper rest helps our bodies to heal, allows for renewal of the body, strengthens the immune system, and lengthens our lifespan. Resting includes more than sleep for physical rest. We also need to rest emotionally, mentally, and spiritually. It is important to take time to relax, such as taking vacations from work and the hustle and bustle of everyday life. Sometimes, we just need to slow down. If we don't do it voluntarily, our bodies have a way of shutting down for us. I'm a witness! Our Creator God rested. Genesis 2:3 (KJV) lets us know that God "rested from all the work of creating that He had done." An example has been left for us.

"O" is for OUTDOORS. While a person may be able to live a few weeks without food and a few days without water, we could only survive a matter of minutes without air. The best air for us to breathe is fresh, outdoors air. Air is composed of oxygen, nitrogen, and a few other gases. We need oxygen to live, and we get that oxygen from the air that we breathe in. It is important for us to get as much fresh air as we can.

However, many of us spend most of our time indoors. We often work inside of a building and then come home where we close the doors and windows and breathe in stale air, odors, and fumes. It important for us to get as much fresh air as we can. Go outside and breathe fresh air daily. Open your windows regularly to allow fresh air to come into your home.

"W" stands for WATER. Can you imagine trying to wash a sink full of dirty dishes in just a cupful of water? On page 190 of the book Health Power, Diehl & Ludington write: "Forcing the body to work with limited amounts of fluid is like trying to wash the dinner dishes in a cupful of water."[5] We can think of drinking water as though we are bathing and cleansing our insides.

Our bodies are 60 to 70 percent water. It is the body's lubricant that helps the rest of the body to work properly. Every aspect of our bodies is affected by not drinking enough water or dehydration. Dehydration affects the normal balance of your body's electrolytes and causes the organs to not function the way they should.

A general rule of thumb for how much water to drink is six to eight cups per day. That equals forty-eight to sixty-four ounces a day. CAUTION: If your health care provider has recommended fluid restrictions for your condition, adjust accordingly!

Water is also important to clean the outside of our bodies. It's helpful for you as well as those you interact with from day to day if you bathe regularly. Not only does water bathe the inside and outside of our bodies to replenish them internally and clean them externally, but hydrotherapy is a great form of treatment for healing.

"N" is for NUTRITION. All the principles I'm sharing are important, but nutrition is a MAJOR player, and probably the area in which we have the most difficulty with self-control. There are so many confusing messages and different "diet plans" and theories. There is a lot of socialization associated with eating. We eat to celebrate most occasions, and the food choices may taste great, but they are often not the best for our health. We grew up eating a certain way, and often those habits can be hard to break, whether bad or good.

The question has been asked, "Do you eat to live, or do you live to eat?" Your response can make a huge difference in your food choices. A popular quote by Hippocrates states: "Let food be thy medicine."

Food is God's method of providing our bodies with the energy needed to carry out its functions. Medical science seems to confirm that God's original diet for mankind provides us with a better chance of avoiding many common diseases such as heart disease, stroke, and some cancers. The nutrients needed to maintain good health are contained in fruits, grains, nuts, and vegetables [whole, plant-based foods]. The optimal diet includes foods in their natural state, as grown and simply prepared, so they are tasty and still retain their nutritious value.

"T" represents TRUST. Trust in God or Divine Power. There are many belief systems to which people subscribe and adhere. My belief is that we were created by a Divine Power as found in the Holy Bible. Genesis 1:27 states: "So God created man in His own image . . ." I like how the psalmist phrases it in Psalm 139:14, when he says, "I praise You because I am fearfully and wonderfully made; Your works are wonderful . . ."

Wow! That make us special. Because God created and loves us, we can trust Him as we pursue holistic health and wellness. Jeremiah 29:11 tells us: " 'For I know the plans I have for you', declares the Lord, 'plans to prosper you and not to harm you, plans to give you hope and a future'."

As we continue to develop our trust in the Creator God for guidance, motivation, and deliverance, we develop the confidence to trust the process of healing and transformation.

"O" is for OPTIMISM. There are three "O's" in CROWN TO SOLE. The second one reminds us to be optimistic and have a positive outlook on life. Years ago, Bobby McFerrin popularized the song, "Don't Worry, Be Happy." The sentiment of the song suggests that in life, we will have trouble, but worrying just makes it double. There is another song that I learned years ago when I was a child. It is titled, "You Can Smile" or "There Are Many Troubles That Will Burst Like Bubbles." I believe it was written by A. H. Ackley. The words are:

> *"There are many troubles that will burst like bubbles,*
> *There are many shadows that will disappear.*
> *If you learn to meet them with a smile to greet them*
> *for a smile is better than a frown or tear.*
> *You can smile when you can't say a word.*
> *You can smile when you cannot be heard.*
> *You can smile when it's cloudy or fair.*
> *You can smile anytime, anywhere."*

There have been times after I was diagnosed with autoimmune disorders that I didn't feel like smiling, but I would remember this song and look at myself in the mirror and smile. It made me feel better just having a smile on my face.

It has been reported that negative emotions and depression can negatively affect the immune system and make us more susceptible to certain diseases. Positive emotional states along with good nutrition and regular exercise can strengthen our immune system. This seems to be supported by the scripture found in Proverbs 17:22: "A merry heart does good like medicine, but a broken spirit dries the bones."

"S" represents SUNLIGHT. We often hear of the dangers associated with exposure to sunlight, such as premature skin aging and wrinkling as well as skin cancer. These warnings should be respected; however, we need appropriate sunlight for its physical and mental benefits. Sunlight exposure is necessary for our bodies to produce vitamin D. It seems that so many people have a Vitamin D deficiency these days. Could it be partially due to lack of sun exposure? Sunlight helps with normalizing our blood pressure, it kills germs, and it boosts the immune system.

The winter months are often associated with gloomy, dreary days and decreased sunshine. Consequently, many of us experience more sad days during the winter. When the springtime rolls around and the sun is shining, we get happy again and feel rejuvenated. Some of the mental benefits of sunlight include less stress, elevated mood, and better rest. I'm one of those who tend to do better emotionally in the spring and summer months. It takes much more effort for me to get outside when it's cold and dreary out.

"O" number three stands for OTHERS. In Acts 20:35(KJV), we read, "In all things I have shown you that . . . we must help the weak and remember . . . it is more blessed to give than to receive." Sometimes, we are the ones who are strong and can bless others. Other times, we may be the weak ones and must humble ourselves to receive the assistance and blessing provided by someone else. Realizing that life is not "all about me" helps us to be unselfish. Giving to others enables us to have a sense of purpose. It takes the focus from ourselves and our problems.

During my time of serious illness, when I was asking others to pray for me, I also had friends and relatives struggling with their own serious health concerns. Instead of focusing just on myself and my problems, it was a blessing to me to be concerned about and assist others. I realize we're all in this life together, and we need others to help us make it. Everybody goes through struggles. No one is immune.

There have been so many people who have poured into me and loved on me when I shared my health challenges. I was used to being the one on the other end and trying to help someone else. Now I needed help. My family and friends have come to my rescue in huge ways. One instance stands out in my mind. I shared it on Facebook along with some pictures as part of keeping people in the loop regarding my journey. I will share the post again here.

10/31/19 **Shoutout to my Sisterfriend:** *I have been wanting to post these pics and a story behind them for several days but every time I would think about it, I would start crying. I love you Ellowyn Young Bell! My husband and I recently traveled to the Christian Book Lovers Retreat in North Carolina. I would likely not have been able to attend if it had not been for Ellowyn and Terrence Dion Brown. I'm still somewhat hesitant about traveling far these days (especially alone). I registered for the event somewhat late because I wasn't sure if I would be able to attend. When Terrence Brown expressed interest in attending, we decided to register. Because I was a little late the host hotel told me the discounted rooms were gone, so I booked at a nearby hotel. Ellowyn suggested I contact the director of the event to see about a room at the host hotel at the discounted rate. I did and the director was able to send me a link that worked for me to get the retreat rate at the host hotel. I was also able to change our airline flights so that we were on the same flights as Ellowyn and Dewayne Bell without much difference in cost.*

There were several events at the retreat in which the participants were separated into groups. Without my knowing it beforehand, Ellowyn had arranged with the director of the event to make sure she and I were in the same group just in case I were to have any challenges she would be there to help me. I didn't find this out until later. The reason these particular pics mean so much is that it demonstrates for me humility and the need to allow others to help you. These pics are from the hat painting party. Several months ago, I developed a slight hand tremor which sometimes makes it difficult doing fine discriminatory skills/ tasks with my hands. I felt like I could be okay with the painting part but wasn't sure about some of the other stuff. I was able to do most of it but when it came to the writing, I knew I probably wouldn't be able to do it to my satisfaction because of the tremor. I thought to just leave off the writing, but "Trust" is my chose theme word for 2019. I chose it even before I became ill. I really wanted to include it on my hat. I humbled myself enough to ask Ellowyn if she would do that part for me- something I normally would have been able to do for myself. She graciously obliged. This hat now represents so much to me and it now sits in my home office – my "she-room". God puts people in our lives to bless us. Sometimes we have to humble ourselves and receive the blessings. I pray that I am a blessing to others. Thank you again Ellowyn! Yes, I cried before posting and while I was writing...you know me.

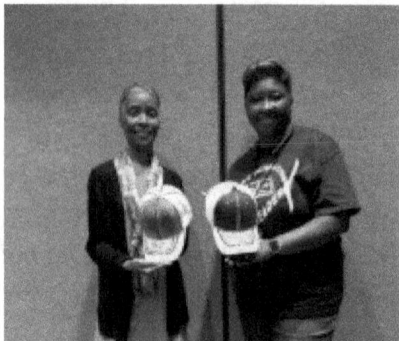

Everyone needs help at some point in their lives. As the song by Joan Baez says: "*No man is an island, no man stands alone. Each man's joy is joy to me, each man's grief is my own. We need one another, so I will defend, each man as my brother, each man as my friend.*"

"L" is for **LOVE**. "And thou shalt love the Lord thy God
with all thy heart, and with all thy soul, and with all
thy mind, and with all thy strength: this is the first
commandment. And the second is like, namely this, Thou
shalt love thy neighbor as thyself. There is none other
commandment greater than these." Mark 12:30,31(KJV)

In plain English, these verses mean that we are to love God with
everything that we have and everything that we are. Don't put
anything or anyone before God. Love other people the way you
love yourself. Treat others the way you want to be treated. That's
not always easy. When we have suffered a tragedy, we sometimes
blame God instead of trusting and loving Him. If we have been
mistreated, it can be difficult to treat the offender with love.
Sometimes, we even have difficulty loving ourselves. However,
when we operate from a place of love, I believe it promotes healing. I like this quote by Peter Abrahams from *The Path of Thunder*;
"You see, love is strong. Stronger than hate even. Love is the only
thing that can kill hate, nothing else. You see, hate destroys and
that's why love is stronger. It builds."[6] I encourage you to love
God. Love yourself. Love others.

I have been so blessed to be surrounded by love on my journey. My
family, friends, church members, coworkers, and even my Facebook friends have contributed to my healing process by loving
on me in so many ways. My husband, Terrence, has truly lived up
to our marriage vows of loving through sickness and in health. He
has been a rock for me. So many times, when I have been fright-
ened, he has calmed me or just listened when that is what I
needed. He shouldered much of responsibilities of the household
that we had previously shared. I began to worry about him and
pray for him because of the added burden on him. But he has taken
it   all   in   stride   and   not   complained.

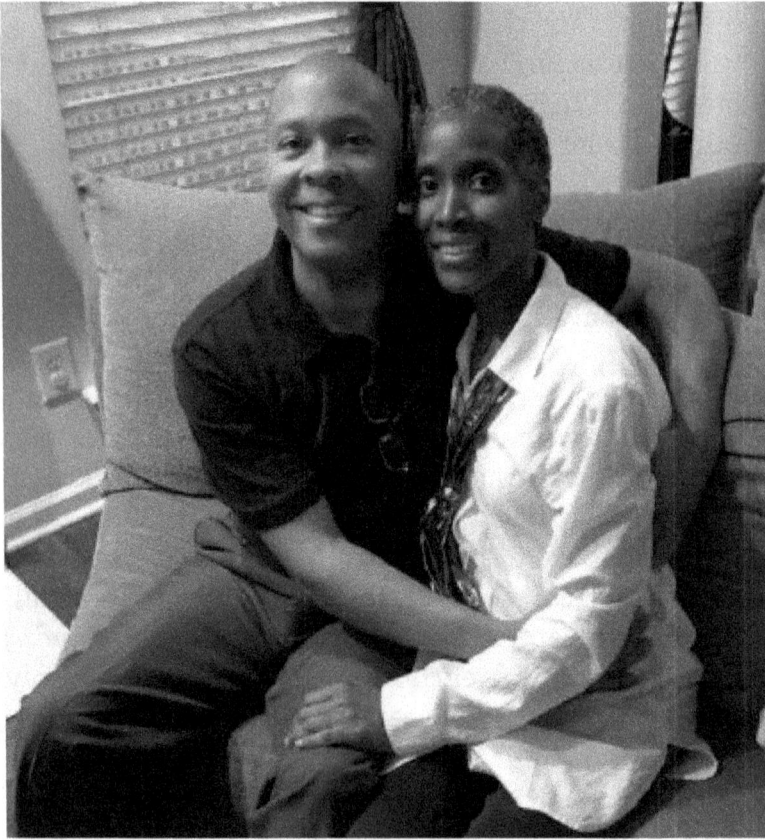

(Terrence and I relaxing at home!)

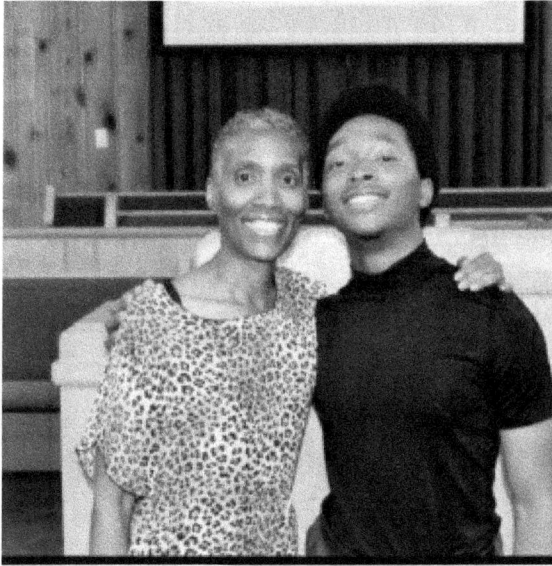

My sons have stepped up to do their part as well. I previously mentioned about my older son and I crying on each other's shoulders as he attempted to console me when I was having a meltdown. I had another very touching experience with my younger son, Jordan, one evening when I was having severe abdominal pain and wasn't sure if I needed to go to the emergency room again. I had already been to the ER for similar pain a couple of months prior. Jordan sensed that I was not doing well and came into the room to check on me. I was pleasantly surprised when he knelt beside the bed and began to pray for me. After the prayer, he made tea for me. Usually I'm the one making tea for him when he is ill. (*My younger son, Jordan, and I in the picture*)

Then there is my mom, Valeria Montague, who at the time I became ill was seventy-nine years old and looking forward to turning eighty. We live about three-and-a-half hours' drive from each other, and she does not drive on the interstate.

When she learned I was ill, she packed a suitcase and found a ride to my home just in case she needed to stay and take care of me. I don't take the people in my life and their love for me for granted. I am grateful and thank God for blessing and loving me.

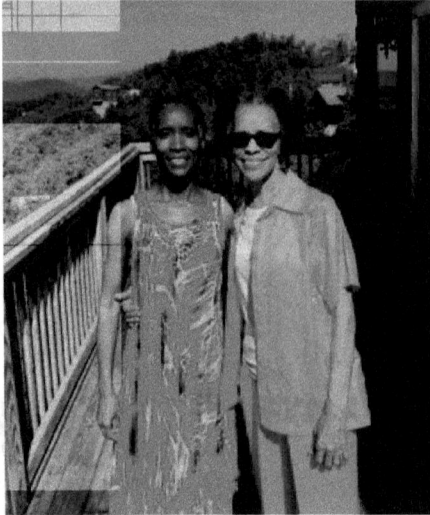

(Mom and I enjoying the sunshine at the
2019 Shields Family Reunion)

"E" stands for **EXERCISE**. "Jesus saith unto him, 'Rise, take up thy bed and walk.' And immediately the man was made whole, and took up his bed, and walked." John 5:6 (KJV) Ah! The lame man's healing came about as a result of his faith, but he also had to act! We don't necessarily have to pick up our bed; however, for optimal health, we do need to get out of the bed after a good night's rest. Make up the bed. Take a walk! It may be that you prefer some other form of physical activity, but I hope you get the point. Get moving. Walking is one of the simplest forms of exercise if you are able and doesn't cost anything. You don't even have to join a gym or anything like that.

Thirty minutes a day of cardiovascular activity is recommended. A brisk walk is an easy and effective way of achieving this. It will do wonders to improve mind and body. Strength training is also important for good muscle tone and bone health. Sometimes it helps to find a partner or group to exercise with to keep you motivated and accountable. Whatever you prefer, just do it.

CHAPTER 15 –
LEARNING FROM
OTHERS

My journey of pursuing holistic wellness is not one that I have undertaken alone or without help. Since I was a child, I have been interested in what I could do to take care of myself. When I was very young, the pastor of my church invited a lady to come and teach the congregation about natural remedies and nutrition. I found the information very interesting, but I overhead several of the adults seeming to make fun of her, perhaps because they didn't want to make some of the changes she was suggesting. Her name was Agatha Thrash, M.D. and I believe she was the founder of Uchee Pines Lifestyle Institute in Alabama. As I grew older, I began to follow her, by attending her seminars and obtaining some of her books so I could learn more. Currently, I often utilize some of the online resources from the Uchee Pines institute. Over the years, I have learned a lot from her teachings and research that I continue to use today, such as hydrotherapy practices, the appropriate use of activated charcoal, nutritional practices, and other natural remedies.

When I was a young adult in college, I met another student, Donna Green, (now Donna Green-Goodman) a young lady who has become a lifelong associate, role model, and mentor as it relates to creating my lifestyle for wellness. Donna was diagnosed with breast cancer over twenty years ago, and largely pursued non-traditional means for treatment of her disease. She tells her story in her book, *Somethin' to Shout About,* recounting how she overhauled her diet and adopted a whole food, plant-based diet in addition to some of the other principles I have described previously.[7] Donna has remained cancer free and continues to share her story. She and her husband, Edward, continue to motivate and teach others how to adopt a healthful lifestyle through their business, Lifestyle Therapeutix.

One of the reasons I appreciate Donna is because she is so down to earth and excited about life. When I was responsible for hosting a wellness seminar back in the 1990s for my church, I knew Donna was the one who could connect with the attendees and encourage them, because of her presentation style. Several years ago, in 2017, Donna hosted an online cooking class. I don't like to cook [as you well know by now] but was interested in preparing more fresh, wholesome dishes, so I registered for the classes. We had a lot of fun, even though part of the time I had to laugh at myself because I didn't always know what I was doing, and my dishes didn't quite look as nice as Donna's. Fast forward to 2019, and the lessons I learned in her class came in handy as I made the choice to try to eliminate processed foods from my diet as much as possible. I still follow Donna online and in person as I strive to continue learning to better myself and improve my abilities to assist others. (Donna and I at Lifestyle Therapeutix)

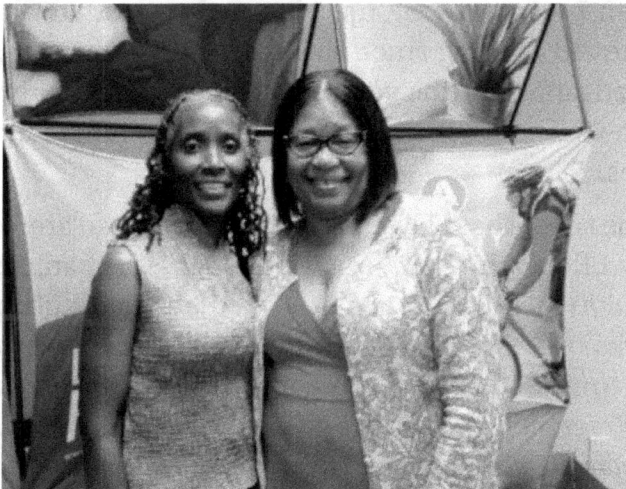

Curtis and Paula Eakins, the husband-and-wife team of Abundant Living TV have also been special role models for me. I had the opportunity to present alongside Paula at a Health Fair years ago during a women's retreat, and we have stayed connected. As part of my growth and learning, I have enjoyed attending wellness seminars that Curtis and Paula host. I am always blessed and encouraged to continue my journey and am better equipped to serve as a result of having learned from them.

In 2011, I attended a series of classes sponsored by Worldwide Medical Missionary Movement. The facilitators were another husband-and-wife team, Jim and Dorcas Ayodo. The classes were comprehensive and included spiritual lessons, nutrition and cooking classes, the use of medicinal plants and herbs, hydrotherapy, and other natural treatments. We had hands-on experience treating clients who came for services. This was an awesome experience, and it was during this time I gained more confidence in using natural treatments on myself and became far less dependent on medications. It was as a result of these classes that I chose to fully adopt a plant-based diet and finally decided to give up fish and dairy products.

Both of my parents were teachers, and we had many books in our home when I was growing up. I learned to read at an early age and have loved reading since the age of four years old. That has not changed, and over the years my home library has grown with health and wellness books in addition to my medical books and other titles.

Some of the titles that I have particularly enjoyed are: *Ministry of Healing* by Ellen White; *Eat to Live* by Joel Fuhrman, M.D.; *Health Power: Healthy by Choice Not Chance* by Aileen Ludington and Hans Diehl; Forks over Knives edited by Gene Stone; *Fighting Disease with Food* compiled by Colleen Louw; *Square One: Healing Cancer Coaching Program Guide Book* by Chris Wark; and *Goodbye Lupus: How a Medical Doctor Healed Herself Naturally With Supermarket*

Foods by Brooke Goldner, M.D. There are many others in my library, but I wanted to share a few.

A couple of documentaries that have been eye-opening and helpful for me are *What the Health*, *Forks Over Knives*, and *Game Changers*. It is important for me to continue learning and improving myself so that I can live my best life and be able to use what I have learned and experienced to bless someone else.

CHAPTER 16 – MY CUSTOMIZED TREATMENT PLAN FOR MY AUTOIMMUNE DISORDERS

Autoimmune disorders are conditions or illnesses in which the body's immune system attacks itself. Normal body tissues are attacked by antibodies that the immune system has manufactured. There are many autoimmune disorders, and inflammation plays a big part in the destructive process. My first goal when I realized I was likely dealing with an autoimmune disorder was to combat the inflammation. I began to research and inquire as to ways I could reduce the inflammation naturally.

A friend of my oldest brother shared with me the ingredients for an anti-inflammatory "green drink." We immediately purchased the recommended ingredients, and I started drinking eight ounces of this "smoothie" twice a day for several months. I believe she may have recommended to juice the ingredients, but since I was not trying to lose weight and needed the fiber, I decided to just mix mine in the blender along with some water. Also, I didn't know where my juicer was at the time, and I remembered that it was hard to clean.

My green drink consists of cucumber, kale, celery, parsley, lemon juice, ginger, and turmeric. Sometimes I use the ginger and turmeric roots, but most of the time I use ginger and turmeric powder. I was not given specific amounts to use, so I just did what I felt. Generally, I will use one cucumber, one or two celery stalks, four or five kale leaves (depending on the leaf size), a handful of parsley, several shakes of the ginger and turmeric powders, and two to four cups of water. Sometimes I add flaxseed or chia seed to increase my healthy fat intake and my omega-3 consumption. These ingredients are blended to a drinkable consistency. I found that I don't like it lumpy. I also add fresh pineapple sometimes to help sweeten the taste. However, when I first started drinking it, I really didn't care what it tasted like if it was going to help me heal.

My next goal was to eliminate from my diet foods and drinks that could cause inflammation. I was already not eating meat or dairy products, but I was still eating processed foods. It was a challenge [and still is] trying to eliminate the processed foods and eat mostly fresh, whole food, plant-based meals. However, I'm trying to live abundantly and thrive, so I keep moving forward. When I go to the grocery store, most of my time is spent in the produce section, and then I move to the section with the dry beans, peas, lentils, and whole grains. My beverage of choice is water, but sometimes I will drink herbal, medicinal teas or make my own juices. I have even started making my own milk. So far, I have only made almond milk, but I have seen recipes for other plant-based milks that I would like to try.

There are so many different fruits and vegetables, and I try to make sure to include all the colors in my diet. Because I don't like to cook, my dishes are simple. I eat a lot of green vegetables [kale, spinach, collard, mustard and turnip greens, and cabbage]. Sweet potatoes, white or red potatoes, and carrots, cucumbers are staples in our house now. I also eat a lot of pinto, black, white, lima, green, and garbanzo beans, black-eyed peas, and lentils. Broccoli is a dish we eat often. Brown/black rice and oatmeal are also easy favorites. We try to keep the pantry stocked with cashews, almonds, pecans, walnuts, dates, raisins. Some of my favorite fruits are apples, oranges, pineapples, grapes, strawberries, blueberries, blackberries, raspberries, watermelon, and bananas. There are many other fresh food selections that we enjoy in addition to the foods I have mentioned.

The weight loss I experienced was a source of concern for me, so I started eating a lot of bananas, avocados, nuts, and potatoes to increase my calories and help me gain weight. It hasn't really helped a lot yet to regain all the pounds lost, but I'm not losing at the rate I was previously and I am feeling much better than I was before.

I received many suggestions for different supplements, but thus far I have not been using a lot of them. The one that I used with some consistency for a period is black seed oil. I would take it internally, but I also started using it on some nodules that I'd developed on my forearms. The nodules were there for several months, and none of my providers knew exactly what they were even after imaging studies were done. My friend, Amy, who is a cancer survivor, suggested I rub the black seed oil over the nodules. They finally went away. I don't know if they went away due to the black seed oil or not, but that was what I used along with moist heat and compression. I also sometimes use herbal teas and essential oils such as lavender, peppermint, and lemon.

When my muscles and bones were severely painful and sore, I would soak in a warm tub of water with Epsom salts. Usually, I use hot to cold showers as my favorite form of hydrotherapy. The hot water feels so good on my muscles and joints. Five to seven minutes of hot water is followed by thirty seconds of cool/cold water. I repeat this for three cycles. It helps to improve the immune system and just feels good. Well, the hot water part feels good; the cold water not so much, but it is part of the process.

As my stamina began to increase and the pain eased, I was able to start again with regular walking exercise. My husband and I began to walk around the neighborhood. Initially, I could only walk a few steps and had to come back into the house. Gradually, I was able to walk the whole circle of the neighborhood at a brisk pace.

Resting is very important for healing, and I try to be very intentional about going to bed at a time that will allow me to get seven to eight hours of sleep. Usually by 9 or 10 p.m., I am heading to bed. In the past, it has been difficult to say no when I am asked to do something; however, I have learned to let some things go and not feel guilty about it. I still like to be active and involved, but I choose to honor my body and give it the rest it needs physically, emotionally, mentally, and spiritually.

Listening to inspirational and meditational music is also a part of my regular habit to help me renew my mind and transform my life.

My self-care routine starts and ends with my mindset rituals. Upon awakening, I thank God for life and for taking care of me through the night. I read scriptures and inspirational devotional passages to help me start my day and get me in the right frame of mind. Sometimes, I'll journal or write out my gratitude. Writing out my gratitude is a practice I was inspired to do by my friend, Irene, whom I met when we were members of Toastmasters International. While I was used to thinking about what I was grateful for, I was impressed that she had started the practice of writing her gratitude daily and had done it for many years. Irene reached out to me after learning I was ill and we were able to go out and enjoy a meal together. (Irene and I dining in the picture)

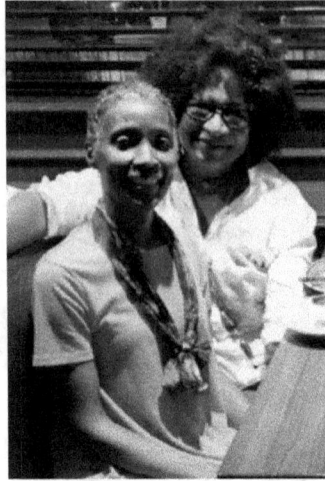

One of the things that really has given me comfort and confidence through this process is my garden. For many years, I had wanted to plant a fruit or vegetable garden, but for some reason was never able to get around to it in the past. It may be that I was just too busy, or more likely it's the fact that I really didn't know what to do, so I was afraid to try. I laugh at myself for waiting until I was sick and could barely move to decide to go ahead and plant a garden. When I asked others what to do or looked online, I became somewhat confused and almost chickened out. However, one day, I just went to the dollar store and bought some seed packets. My husband and son cleared a spot in the backyard for the garden, and I planted cucumber, kale, lettuce, carrots, and peas. My fear was that nothing would grow. If I could just get even one plant that I could eat, I would consider that a success.

Caring for the garden helped me to get fresh air and exercise in addition to teaching me some life lessons. It was so exciting to watch the plantings go through the process of starting from seeds to developing leaves, becoming small plants, and then the full product ready for harvest. It was a thrill to see my cucumbers, kale, and other vegetables ripen, and I was proud to eat food from my garden. I learned that the process of going from seed to harvest takes time and proper nurturing. Although I call it my garden, I was not alone in caring for it. My husband, brother, and son all took part in helping prepare the ground, water, and weed. Just like in life, we are not alone and need help. I saw my own growth and healing process in lessons learned from the garden. One day, as I was tending the garden, I reflected that just like how the garden grew because of a series of steps including preparing the ground, planting, watering, and weeding; God was showing me that was what He was doing with me. While I was praying for the instantaneous and miraculous healing, I imagined God saying to me, "Karla, I'm taking you through a process, but I've got you baby girl. Just trust me."

My treatment plan and healing are works in progress. As I continue to research and learn more, I try to implement processes that will help me heal. Sometimes I am not as consistent as I would like to be with some areas of self-care. Initially I was very diligent about making and drinking that green drink. After some months went by, I didn't always feel like making it, so I would miss some days. I have tried to get back to a regular routine. The cold weather hampered my walking efforts, but I still try to get it done. One of the things I'm having the most difficulty with is my strength-training routine. I'm not trying to be a power lifting competitor or anything like that, but I do want to get my muscle tone back. Prior to becoming ill, I had developed a strength-training routine, but since the illness, I have not been consistent at all with the training. I'm not going to give up though. Each day is a new day to get it right.

For the most part, I am still medication free. For full transparency though, I will say that when I was having severe abdominal pain and vomiting recently, I finally went to the emergency room. They gave me some medication and I didn't refuse it. I did tell them to give me a pediatric dose, because I was afraid of having a bad reaction. There have been at least one or two times since then that I have had to take the medication for abdominal spasm, because it was so severe, and if I have to, I will take cough drops to calm an uncontrollable cough when other methods are not working. However, I am not on any chronic medications at this point, and I believe it is largely because of the other methods of treatment I have adopted. My goal is to regain my health and remain largely medication free for as long as possible.

PHOTO ALBUM

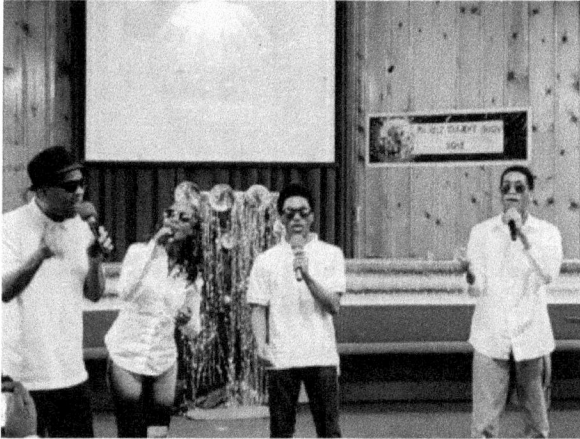

January 2019 (Family Talent Show)
I was beginning to feel the effects of illness but didn't realize I was sick.

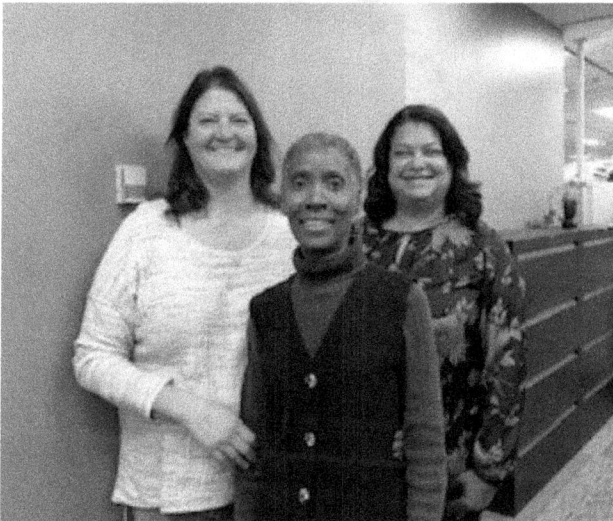

I'm here at work with my colleagues, Dr. Rebecca (Becky) and
Dr. Glenda, who have supported me on this journey.

Thankfully, I was able to attend my sons' performances in February of 2019. Justin was the music director. Jordan was one of the actors

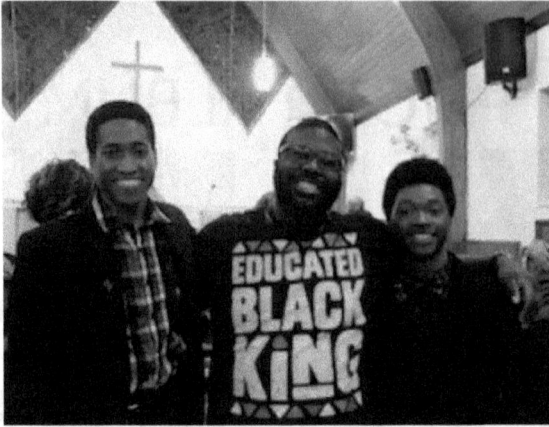

Justin and Jordan with "Chapter 2" director, Alan Nettles

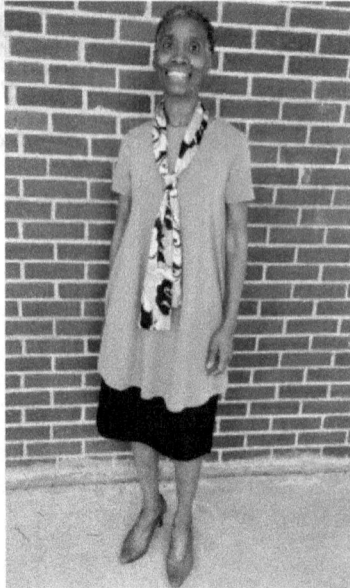

Finally, after a few months, I was able to wear "real" shoes again!

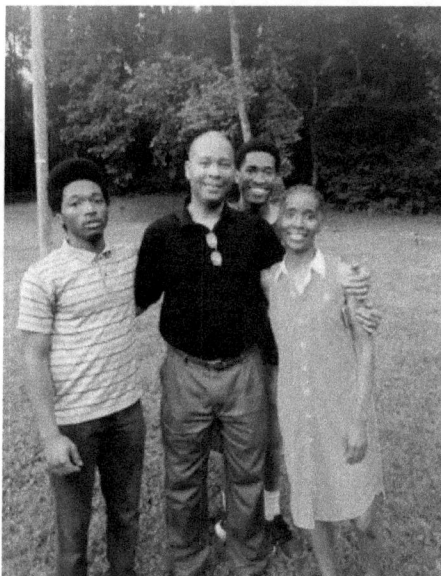

Terrence, Justin, Jordan, and I at the 2019 Family Campbell Reunion

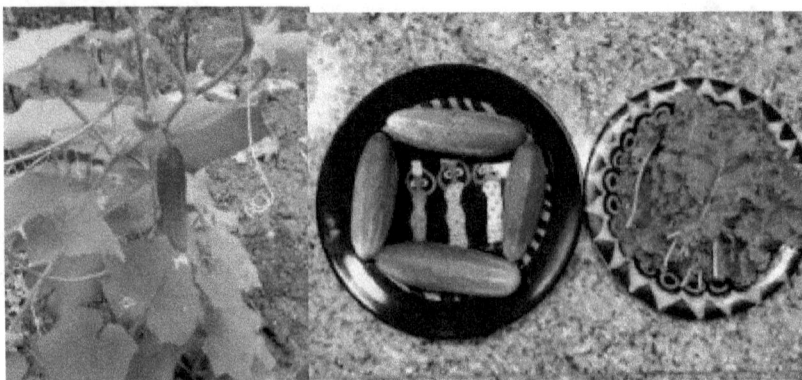

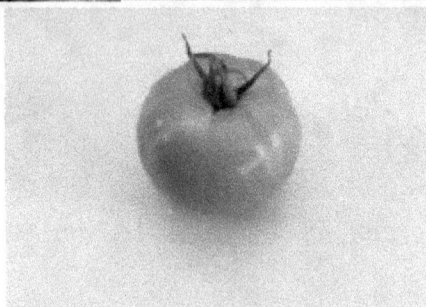

My garden and harvest!

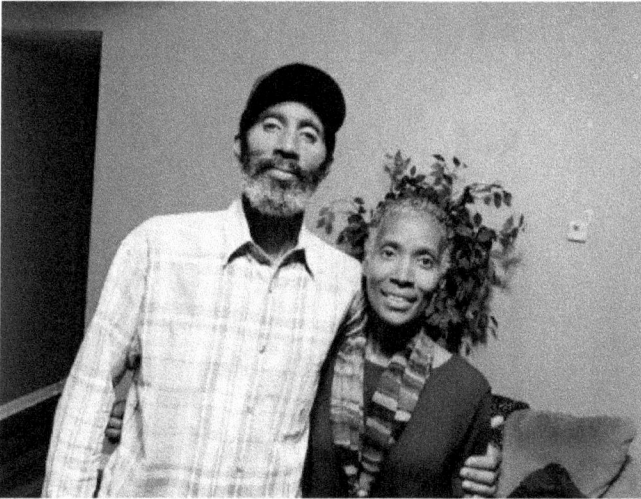

Spending time with my older brother, Glenn, who helped me with my garden.

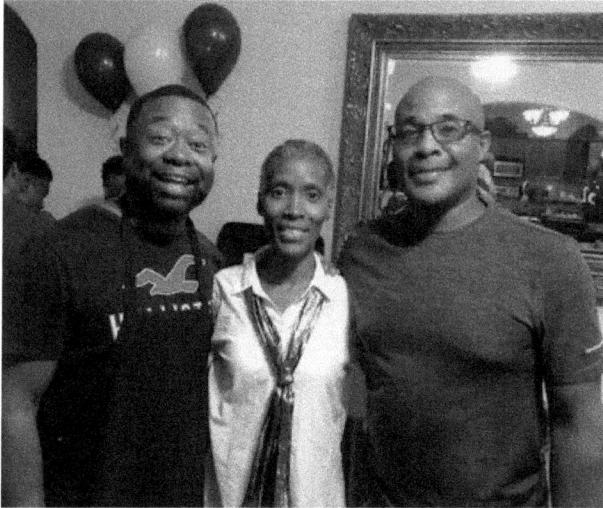

Hanging out and celebrating with my younger brothers, Dewayne and Kevin

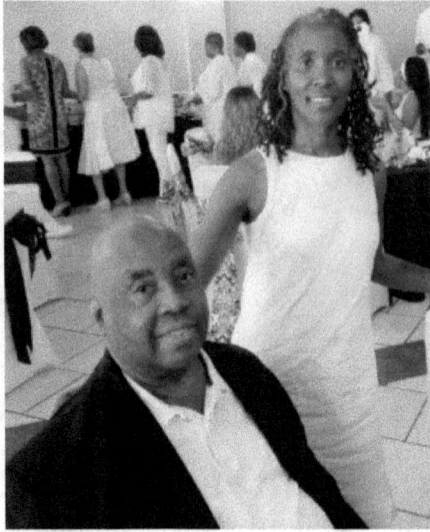

Remembering my dad, Dr. Arnett Montague

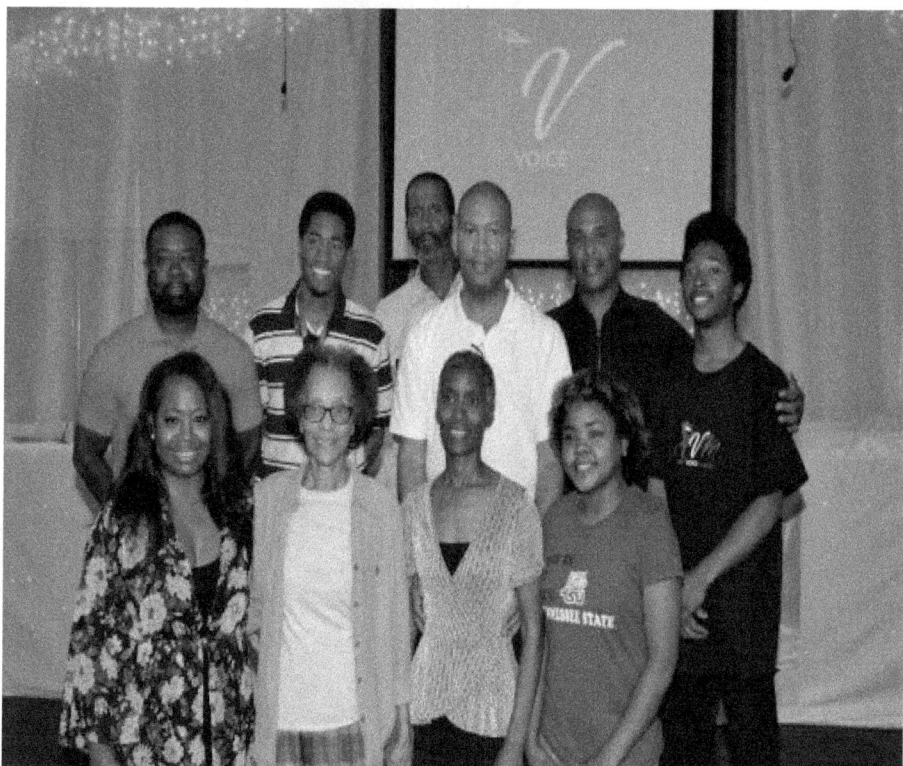

My family showed up for the "My Journey" speaking engagement!

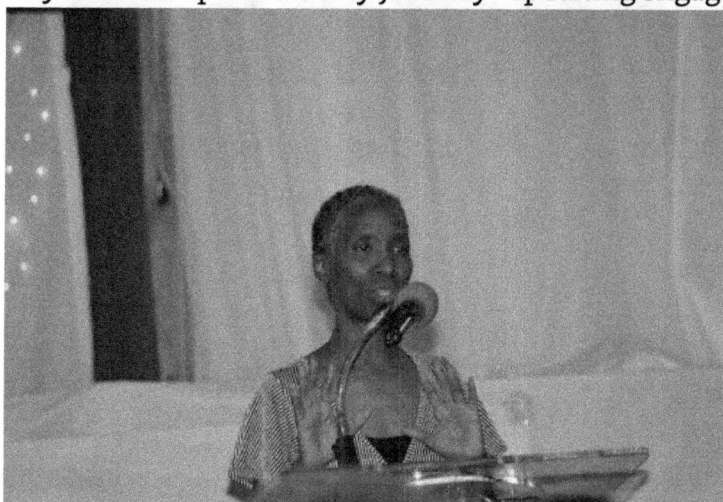

Sharing My Journey 2019

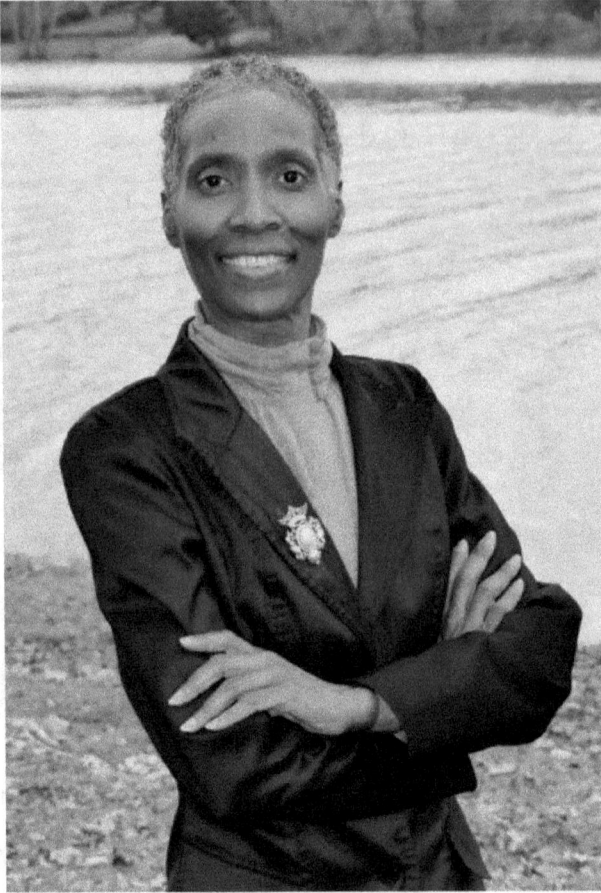

One-year post diagnoses and I'm much better.
"I will bless the Lord at all times. His Praise shall continually
be in my mouth." Psalm 34:1

CONCLUSION

My personal and professional experiences have given me the desire to do my part to encourage and motivate others toward healthful living by providing practical strategies. When I became ill in early 2019 and prayed for healing, I was hoping for a miraculous healing that would occur instantaneously. I wanted to be well even before discovering what was wrong. I told God that when He healed me, I would testify about my healing and give Him the glory. After a while of praying, when I was still sick, I realized that my healing process may take a lot longer than I wanted or that the healing may not look like what I'd expected. *What if God doesn't heal me?* I wondered, or *What if it takes a long time?* I figured I couldn't wait to give God praise and share my story. I needed to praise Him during the challenges and share the blessings along the way.

Many times, we keep our struggles and testimonies of praise to ourselves for various reasons. I have been blessed by others who have shared their stories of challenge and victory, and I'm grateful they have been willing to become transparent and vulnerable enough to share.

Prior to 2019, I had dreams of writing a book to help others transform their lives and create lifestyles of optimal wellness. I had some ideas of how I wanted the book to go, but after I became ill, I began journaling my experience and my book idea changed. My illness also forced me to stop procrastinating and just do it. It's funny how becoming real with your mortality will have you re-evaluating your situation and making changes. Hopefully, I'm making changes for the good that will leave a lasting and positive legacy. I'm learning to not be afraid to pursue dreams and goals. Tomorrow is not promised, so I'm trying to do what I can now.

My journaling prompted me to share my experience in a book that could be an encouragement to someone else. That is what I have prayed about through this book-writing process, and it is my prayer that you have been encouraged. I did not write this book to just talk about myself. Hopefully, my story will encourage, empower, and equip you to take control of your life to live abundantly by God's power. I'm reminded of this quote from Ellen White in the book *Counsels on Health:*

"When we do all we can on our part to have health, then may we expect that the blessed result will follow, and we can ask God in faith to bless our efforts for the preservation of health." [8]

This book does not include everything related to achieving wellness. It is presented as a testimonial of my experience and some of the principles that I have adopted in pursuing wellness and overcoming my autoimmune disorders. It is not meant to take the place of your physician's or health care provider's advice and/or medical treatments. The information presented includes some healthful lifestyle strategies to help you start developing habits to improve your health.

No matter what you have been through or what someone else may have led you to believe, you are of Royalty. You are precious and were created to have dominion over the rest of God's creatures. As you incorporate some of the principles as discussed in Chapter 14, expect to see great benefits as you move toward optimal health and wellness from the **CROWN** of your head **TO** the **SOLE** of your foot! May God direct and bless your efforts.

THANK YOU! I am so grateful to you for reading my book. I would love to hear your feedback and how this book may have benefited you. My goal is to continue to improve so that I can be of greater service.

Please let me know what you thought of the book by leaving a helpful review on Amazon. Thank you so much!

FREE THANK YOU GIFT!

Here is the web address to download a Free Copy of my CROWN TO SOLE Wellness Action Guide and to become a part of my Crown To Sole Wellness community.

https://bit.ly/C2Sactionguide

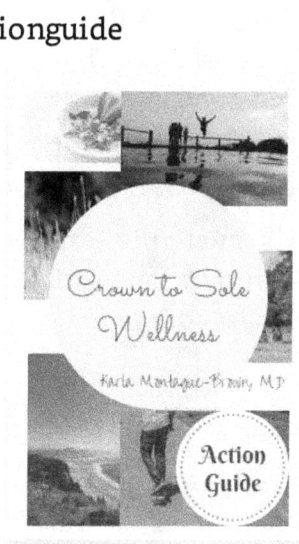

ABOUT THE AUTHOR

Karla Montague-Brown, M.D. has enjoyed many years of experience as a Family Medicine Physician and medical consultant. She is a sought-after speaker and seminar/workshop presenter who is passionate about encouraging, empowering, and equipping individuals to adopt practical lifestyle strategies for pursuing holistic health and wellness.

Her life is enhanced by her husband, Terrence, and the couple enjoys being the parents of two young adult sons, Justin and Jordan.

Dr. Montague-Brown is available for speaking engagements, health and wellness seminars or workshops, retreat presentations, and personal wellness coaching.

Contact information:

Email: KarlaMBrown@crowntosolewellness.com

Website: http://crowntosolewellness.com

Follow on:
Facebook.com/karlamontaguebrownmd
Instagram@karlamontaguebrown
LinkedIn@Karla Montague-Brown, MD
Twitter@KarlaMBrownMD

If you are ready to gain the victory over your chronic auto-immune illness, please schedule a *FREE* Discovery Call with Dr. Montague-Brown at: www.calendly.com/karlambrown to determine if and how she can help you!

REFERENCES

1. Goldner, Brooke. (2015). Goodbye Lupus: How a Medical Doctor Healed Herself Naturally With Supermarket Foods. Austin, TX: Express Results

2. Young, Sarah. (2012). Jesus Today. Nashville, TN: Thomas Nelson

3. Story of Hezekiah in the Holy Bible- 2 Kings Chapter 20

4. White, Ellen. (1905-orig.) (1990-later). The Ministry of Healing (orig.) Ministry of Healing: Health and Happiness (later). Silver Springs, MD: Better Living Publications

5. Diehl, Hans., Ludington, Aileen. (2011). Health Power: Healthy By Choice, Not By Chance! Hagerstown, MD: Review and Herald

6. Abrahams, Peter. (1984). The Path of Thunder. Claremont, Western Cape, South Africa: David Philip Publishers

7. Green-Goodman, Donna. (1999). Somethin' to Shout About, Coldwater, MI: Remnant Publications

8. White, Ellen. (1923). Counsels on Health. Mountain View, CA: Pacific Press (Ch. 59.1)